ALCOHOL AND DRUG ABUSE

METHAMPHETAMINES: ABUSE, HEALTH EFFECTS AND TREATMENT OPTIONS

ALCOHOL AND DRUG ABUSE

Additional books in this series can be found on Nova's website under the Series tab.

Additional E-books in this series can be found on Nova's website under the E-books tab.

ALCOHOL AND DRUG ABUSE

METHAMPHETAMINES: ABUSE, HEALTH EFFECTS AND TREATMENT OPTIONS

JÖRG ORNOY
AND
XIAOLING HE
EDITORS

Nova Science Publishers, Inc.
New York

For permission to use material from this book please contact us:
Telephone 631-231-7269; Fax 631-231-8175
Web Site: http://www.novapublishers.com

Library of Congress Cataloging-in-Publication Data

Methamphetamines : abuse, health effects, and treatment options / editors, Jvrg Ornoy and Xiaoling He.
p. ; cm.
Includes bibliographical references and index.
ISBN 978-1-62100-244-4 (hardcover)
I. Ornoy, Jvrg. II. He, Xiaoling, 1968-
[DNLM: 1. Amphetamine-Related Disorders. 2. Methamphetamine. WM 275]
LC classification not assigned
616.86'4--dc23

2011034213

Published by Nova Science Publishers, Inc. ✝ New York

CONTENTS

PREFACE

Methamphetamine abuse is a significant problem in the United States. It is used by nearly 530,000 Americans ages 12 and older, but the effects are devastating to family and friends of addicts. In this book, the authors present topical research on the abuse, health effects and treatment options of methamphetamine. Some of the topics discussed include the effects of methamphetamine exposure during brain development on cognition and markers of cognitive function; what rodent activity can tell us about methamphetamine abuse; sigma receptors as a potential target for methamphetamine abuse and dependence and methods for confirmatory analysis of methamphetamine in biological samples.

Chapter 1 - Methamphetamine (MA) use among pregnant women is concerning as exposure to MA during brain development increases the risk of short- and long-term detrimental effects, including being born small for gestational age and the risk of being born with birth defects. MA exposure is also associated with increased physiological stress, decreased arousal, and poor quality of movement during the first five days of life. In addition to these relative short-term effects, MA has persistent and long-term effects on cognition in childhood and adolescence, including cognitive impairments in visual motor integration and hippocampus-dependent learning and memory. School performance is delayed and physical ability impaired in MA-exposed children. Consistent with hippocampal dysfunction, children exposed *in utero* to MA have a smaller hippocampus. To increase the authors' understanding of the effects of MA in adolescence and adulthood on brain function, and in particular hippocampal function at these stages of life, translational animal models are helpful. They allow for controlled environmental exposure conditions not feasible in the context of MA exposure in humans. In this chapter, authors will review the human and animal data describing the long-term effects of MA exposure during brain development and illustrate the potential role of altered histaminergic and cholinergic neurotransmitter systems in these effects.

Chapter 2 - Many abused drugs--including methamphetamine--produce a transient and dose-dependent change in locomotor behavior in rodents. Investigators can design experiments where methamphetamine is administered to rodents and locomotor behavior is observed, measured and analyzed, and many researchers have used this behavioral model to investigate the biological basis of methamphetamine's pharmacological activities. Moreover, several theories have been proposed to link locomotor activity findings in rodents to drug abuse and dependence in humans. This paper provides an overview of the theoretical basis of locomotor behavior as a model of human drug abuse and dependence, a critical comment on the methodological variables to be manipulated in a methamphetamine locomotor activity study, and a review of findings on the impact of multiple biological targets on methamphetamine-induced changes in locomotor behavior.

Chapter 3 - Sigma receptors have been identified as two subtypes—σ1 and σ2—and are located throughout the brain. The receptors regulate intraneuronal signaling pathways and a number of ligands have been developed to study the receptors' roles in behavior. Several lines of research indicate that σ1 sigma receptor antagonists decrease the behavioral effects of cocaine, and these ligands have been considered potential stimulant addiction pharmacotherapies. An emerging line of research suggests that σ1 and/or σ2 sigma receptors could play a role in the behavioral effects of methamphetamine. Methamphetamine binds to sigma receptors, and receptor ligands alter the effects of methamphetamine on locomotor behavior in rodents and on dopamine release from neurons. In this chapter, authors provide an overview of sigma receptor pharmacology and summarize findings on the interactions between sigma receptor ligands and cocaine, as well as with methamphetamine's *in vitro* and behavioral effects.

Chapter 4 - Methamphetamine is the most common amphetamine used and, along with 3,4-methylenedioxymethamphetamine (MDMA, Ecstasy), is considered part of a worldwide drug epidemic. Monitoring methamphetamine levels in the body is important for purposes of drug screening for employment, criminal investigations, and therapeutic drug monitoring. While methamphetamine is suitable for detection using immunoassay techniques, these methods tend to have significant cross reactivity with other compounds. Over the last decade, more than eighty different quantitative, confirmatory analytical methods for measuring methamphetamine in biological samples have been published in the scientific literature. Analytical instrumentation used in these methods includes gas chromatography – mass spectrometry (GC-MS), liquid chromatography – mass spectrometry (LC-MS), capillary electrophoresis (CE), among others. These assays are capable of quantifying methamphetamine concentrations in a variety of biological matrices, including blood, plasma, urine, hair, and fingernails. Some of these techniques can achieve detection as low as 0.1 ng/mL (1 ppb) concentrations. The strengths and limitations of these methodologies will be discussed in the context of methamphetamine analysis. Additionally, methods that can simultaneously measure methamphetamine levels as well as metabolites and other drugs of abuse will be highlighted.

Chapter 5 - Authors investigated whether pretreatment with isoliquiritigenin (ISL), an anti-oxidant flavonoid obtained from *Glycyrrhizae* species, affected methamphetamine (METH)-induced hyperlocomotion, conditioned place preference (CPP), and stereotypy in mice. Pretreatment of male ICR mice with ISL (20 mg/kg, i.p.) significantly inhibited METH (1 mg/kg, i.p.)-induced hyperlocomotion compared with that of vehicle-pretreated subjects, but there were no significant alterations in the tissue levels of monoamines and their metabolites in the cerebral cortex, the region of striatum and nucleus accumbens, and the region of thalamus and hypothalamus between mice with and without ISL pretreatment. Mice treated with ISL prior to METH (0.5 mg/kg) preconditioning showed a significant METH-induced CPP, similar to that observed in mice treated with vehicle prior to METH preconditioning. The total incidence of METH (10 mg/kg)-induced stereotypy was unaffected by pretreatment with ISL. These observations suggest that ISL selectively inhibits METH-induced hyperlocomotion in mice.

Chapter 6 – Background: Gender differences in substance abusing populations have been examined, with some drug treatment strategies found to be more successful for women than for men. Although the female adult cocaine-using population has been well characterized, less is known about the characteristics of the female adult methamphetamine (MA) user. Objective: To determine the similarities and differences between MA- and cocaine-dependent pregnant and parenting women. Design: Authors conducted a retrospective review of women enrolled in the Stork Club, an outpatient drug treatment program for pregnant and parenting women (n=202). Demographics, drug use history, education/employment status prior to treatment, and treatment discharge information were obtained from medical chart reviews using the Los Angeles County Participant Registration Reporting System. Psychiatric symptomatology was assessed using the Psychosocial Assessment

Questionnaire. Continuous variables were analyzed using two-tailed t-tests and categorical variables with chi-square tests. Significance was accepted at $P<0.05$. Results: The cocaine-using women (n=100) were more likely to be homeless (P=0.003), recipients of public assistance (P= 0.03), engage in criminal activity during treatment (P=0.0001), consume alcohol (P=0.02) and drop out of treatment after unsatisfactory progress (P=0.03). In contrast, the MA-using women (n=102) were more likely to successfully complete the treatment program (P=0.02) and own a vehicle (P=0.03); however they were more likely to have contact with intravenous drug users (P=0.01), use a needle within the past year (P=0.01), and use drugs more than once per day at discharge (P=0.01) than the cocaine-using women. Both substance abusing groups had a high incidence of mood disorders. There were no differences in the incidence or types of psychiatric symptomatology between the groups. Discussion: These findings suggest there are significant differences between MA- and cocaine-using women, with MA-using women facing fewer social barriers. However MA-using women are potentially higher risk for Hepatitis C and HIV due to an increased likelihood of exposure to intravenous drug use. Implications of the authors' findings include the benefits of tailoring treatment and prevention programs to specific substances of abuse.

Chapter 7 - Methamphetamine is a dangerous psychostimulant because of its high abuse potential and neurotoxic effects. This stimulant drug alters neurotransmitter storage, release and recycling in the central nervous system and increases levels of extraneuronal dopamine. The dopamine release is caused by methamphetamine's actions at the neuronal membrane-bound dopamine transporter and at the intraneuronal vesicular monoamine transporter. An understanding of how these monoamine transporters function and their interactions with methamphetamine to cause dopamine release is important to understand the pyschostimulant's behavioral and neurotoxic effects.

Chapter 8- Methamphetamine (METH) and amphetamine (AMPH) are known to cause various behavioral changes, such as increased locomotor activity, stereotypy and prepulse inhibition (PPI) disruption, not only in humans but also in rodents. These behavioral changes are caused by releasing dopamine (DA), serotonin (5-HT) and noradrenaline (NA) within the brain. *p*-Hydroxyamphetamine (*p*-OHA), an active metabolite of both METH and AMPH, also has a number of pharmacological actions similar to those induced by drugs of abuse. Peripherally metabolized *p*-OHA does not easily cross the blood-brain barrier, but centrally metabolized *p*-OHA results in long-lasting stimulant effects. For example, intracerebroventricular administration of *p*-

OHA induces a head-twitch response, indicating the involvement of the central serotonergic system. Also, *p*-OHA induces increased locomotor activity, indicating the involvement of the dopaminergic system. Moreover, *p*-OHA causes PPI disruption, indicating the involvement of the dopaminergic, serotonergic and noradrenergic systems. In in vitro experiments, *p*-OHA inhibits monoamine oxidase type A (MAO-A), thereby eliciting an increase in DA, NA and 5-HT levels. In this paper, authors review the pharmacological properties and probable mechanisms of action of *p*-OHA.

Chapter 9 - Since the early 1950s, Japan has experienced three major epidemics of methamphetamine (METH) use. Increasing prevalence rates in the general population for METH use have recently been reported from other pan-pacific nations. METH use disorder still imposes a burden on current mental health in Japan. Strong cravings are a feature of METH use disorder, as many patients find difficulty in refraining from re-using it during abstinence. Recent functional neuroimaging studies show that the craving for METH may be associated with reduced activity in some brain areas involved in decision making. Most noticeably, the paranoid-hallucinatory state resembling paranoid schizophrenia has been regarded as a hallmark of METH-induced psychosis. The current diagnosis of substance-induced psychotic disorder is defined by DSM-IV as a prototypical intoxication-induced or withdrawal-associated psychotic episode. Even the substance-induced psychotic disorder that occurs in the context of substance use disorder has not been sufficiently recognized. Although METH-induced psychosis usually resolves rapidly with the cessation of stimulant use, a subset of currently abstinent METH-dependent patients develop protracted psychosis even after long-term abstinence. Several reports indicate that protracted METH psychosis is more likely to occur among METH abusers with a pre-morbid schizoid/schizotypal personality trait and those with a family history of schizophrenia among first-degree relatives. Further study is needed concerning the role of pre-morbid vulnerability to protracted METH psychosis. Recent studies have also noted a high rate of the life time prevalence of affective symptoms such as depression, suicide attempts, and impulsivity in METH abusers. Caution should be exercised in treating female METH abusers who have a higher risk of suicide than male METH abusers. Studies using positron emission tomography demonstrated that exposure to METH induces a robust change in the neurotransmission of dopamine and serotonin neurons. These studies have shown that the reductions of dopamine and serotonin transporter are associated with cognitive impairment and enhanced impulsivity in patients with METH-induced psychosis.

In: Methamphetamines
Editors: J. Ornoy and X. He
ISBN: 978-1-62100-244-4

Chapter 1

THE EFFECTS OF METHAMPHETAMINE EXPOSURE DURING BRAIN DEVELOPMENT ON COGNITION AND MARKERS OF COGNITIVE FUNCTION

***Jessica A. Siegel*[1] *and Jacob Raber*[1,2,3]**

[1]Department of Behavioral Neuroscience, Oregon Health and Science University, Portland, OR, US

[2]Department of Neurology, Oregon Health and Science University, Portland, OR, US

[3]Division of Neuroscience, Oregon National Primate Research Center, Beaverton, OR, US

ABSTRACT

Methamphetamine (MA) use among pregnant women is concerning as exposure to MA during brain development increases the risk of short- and long-term detrimental effects, including being born small for gestational age and the risk of being born with birth defects. MA exposure is also associated with increased physiological stress, decreased arousal, and poor quality of movement during the first five days of life. In addition to these relative short-term effects, MA has persistent and long-term effects on cognition in childhood and adolescence, including cognitive impairments in visual motor integration and hippocampus-dependent learning and memory. School performance is delayed and physical ability impaired in MA-exposed children. Consistent with hippocampal dysfunction, children exposed *in utero* to MA have a smaller hippocampus. To increase our understanding of the effects of MA in adolescence and adulthood on brain function, and in particular hippocampal function at these stages of life, translational animal models are helpful. They allow for controlled environmental exposure conditions not feasible in the context of MA exposure in humans. In this chapter, we will review the human and animal data describing the long-term effects of MA exposure during brain development and illustrate the potential role of altered histaminergic and cholinergic neurotransmitter systems in these effects.

INTRODUCTION

In this chapter, we will focus on the long-term effects of methamphetamine (MA) exposure during brain development on brain function later in life. MA is a highly addictive central nervous system psychomotor stimulant. In the United States, MA became popular in the 1940s when it was administered to World War II soldiers to promote wakefulness and prevent fatigue, effects that are common among all psychomotor stimulants (Gilman, Rall, Nies, & Taylor, 1993; Gonzales, Mooney, & Rawson, 2010). Production and use of MA for non-medical purposes began to rise in the 1960s and in response to this increase MA was eventually classified as a Schedule II drug by the United States Drug Enforcement Administration (Gettig, Grady, & Nowosadzka, 2006; Gonzales et al., 2010; NIDA, 2010).

MA has a high abuse potential compared to other psychomotor stimulants, likely due in part to its long half-life, its high lipid solubility making transfer across the blood-brain barrier relatively easy, and the fact that MA is metabolized into another active psychomotor stimulant, amphetamine (AMPH), prior to excretion (Barr et al., 2006; Cruickshank & Dyer, 2009; Good, Solt, Acuna, Rotmensch, & Kim, 2010). The prevalence of MA abuse is also likely due in part to the wide availability of the precursors, such as pseudoephedrine, and its ease of manufacture (Gonzales et al., 2010; Sulzer, Sonders, Poulsen, & Galli, 2005). In 2005, the Combat Methamphetamine Epidemic Act was passed, placing federal regulations on the sale of pseudoephedrine (DEA, 2006; Gonzales et al., 2010). Despite a reduction in "mom and pop" meth labs, the use and abuse of MA continues to be a problem.

While recent data suggest an overall decline in MA use in the United States in recent years (NSDUH, 2007), not all epidemiological data show this decrease. Emergency department visits for MA-related issues, for example, increased over 50% from 1995 to 2002 (NIDA, 2006). Similarly, the number of individuals admitted to drug abuse treatment centers for MA addiction increased substantially from 1992 to 2004 (DASIS, 2008; NIDA, 2006). MA use has historically been localized to the rural western portion of the United States (DASIS, 2008; NSDUH, 2007). In more recent years, however, use of the drug has spread across the country (NIDA, 2006).

Adult MA use has effects on learning, memory, and executive function (for a review, see Cruickshank & Dyer, 2009; Scott et al., 2007). For example, adults who used MA for an average of 10.5 years show deficits on a word-recall memory task (Thompson et al., 2004) while use for an average of 30 months results in impaired memory and greater impulsivity on a delayed-discounting task (Hoffman et al., 2006). However, not all studies find such pronounced cognitive impairments in MA abusers, albeit cognitive function is consistently lower than that of non-users (Johanson et al., 2006).

Use of MA by Women of Childbearing Age

Compared to other drugs of abuse, MA use among women is abnormally high (DAWN, 2010) and MA use increases the likelihood of engaging in risky sexual behavior, thereby increasing the chance of a female MA user becoming pregnant (Zule, Costenbader, Meyer, & Wechsberg, 2007). Fetuses are at high risk of MA exposure since most MA-using women are of child-bearing age and MA use is the most common reason for pregnant women to seek drug counseling (Little, Snell, & Gilstrap, 1988; Terplan, Smith, Kozloski, & Pollack, 2009). In 2008, 23.7% of emergency department visits involving MA-related issues were made by patients between the ages of 18 and 24 while 34.7% of visits were made by patients between the ages of 25 and 34 (DAWN, 2010). In 2009, the average age of initiating MA use was 19.3 years (NSDUH, 2009). MA use in the 1980's and 90's was generally confined to Caucasian men driving trucks, working construction, or performing other physically demanding jobs. However, the demographic profile of MA use has widened to other populations, including women (Gonzales et al., 2010). According to the National Survey on Drug Use and Health, women make up 45% of individuals admitted to drug abuse treatment centers for MA abuse in the United States. In contrast, women make up only 26% of individuals admitted to drug abuse treatment centers for alcohol or marijuana abuse (DASIS, 2008; NSDUH, 2007). Due to this increase prevalence of MA use among pregnant women, the number of children exposed to MA *in utero* increased over the past two decades (Terplan et al., 2009).

Maternal MA use is associated with increased risk of preterm birth, complications associated with hypertension, placental abruption, physical abnormalities at birth (Good et al., 2010; Smith et al., 2008), as well as cognitive impairments (Chang et al., 2009; Chang et al., 2004; Piper et al., 2011). Infants exposed to MA or MA and AMPH during pregnancy show reduced visual recognition in the Fagan Test of Infant Intelligence (Struthers & Hansen, 1992). Heavy MA use at any point during pregnancy is also associated with lower arousal, increased lethargy, and physiological stress during the first 5 days of life. MA exposure during the third trimester is specifically associated with poor movement quality (Paz et al., 2009; Smith et al., 2008).

The effects of MA exposure during brain development persist into childhood and adolescence. Heavy MA use at any point during pregnancy is associated with poor motor ability, as measured by grasping, at 1 year of age. However this impairment is gone by 3 years (Smith et al., 2011). MA exposure results in impaired visual motor integration, attention, and verbal memory in 3-16 year old children, and these impairments are associated with reduced hippocampal, putamen, and globus pallidus volumes (Chang et al., 2004). MA exposure during any point of pregnancy also impairs visual motor integration in 3-4 year old children (Chang et al., 2009). MA-exposed children show impairments in hippocampus-dependent spatial memory at 7-9 years of age, but no effects are found on other cognitive tasks, including intelligence quotient and visual-spatial working memory (Piper et al., 2011). MA-exposed children are also more likely to be behind in school, diagnosed with Attention Deficit Hyperactivity Disorder, and to show pronounced problems in executive function as assessed by parental ratings on the Behavioral Rating Inventory of Executive Function questionnaire compared to unexposed children (Piper et al., 2011). Following children exposed to AMPH and/or MA to the age of 14, MA/AMPH exposure was associated with reductions in intelligence quotient, impairments in school performance due to delays in math and language development, and impairments in physical ability (for a review, see Lester & Lagasse, 2010).

Children exposed to both MA and alcohol *in utero* show reduced striatal volumes that are correlated with cognitive deficits measured by the full-scale intelligence quotient compared to children exposed only to alcohol (Sowell et al., 2010). MA/alcohol-exposed children also show more diffuse brain activation during a word recall task compared to children exposed only to alcohol. There might be a compensatory enhancement in brain activation in MA-exposed children to support impaired recall on a word memory task and a weaker verbal memory network (Lu et al., 2009).

Although there are consistent effects of MA exposure during brain development on cognition, there are individual differences in the degree of these impairments. For example, despite overall group differences between MA-exposed and unexposed children, some MA-exposed children are rated on the Behavior Rating Inventory of Executive Function and perform in a test of spatial memory similar to unexposed children (Piper et al., 2011). Individual differences in the degree of cognitive impairment after MA exposure suggest that other factors, such as genetic factors, may modulate the susceptibility to develop cognitive impairment after *in utero* MA exposure. Women who use MA during pregnancy often also drink alcohol, smoke and use other recreational drugs. Because of this polydrug use, MA-specific effects are difficult to study in humans and thus controlled MA exposure experiments using animal models are pertinent.

Rodent Models to Study the Long-term Effects of MA Exposure during Brain Development on Hippocampal Function

The hippocampus is an area of the brain that is important for many aspects of cognitive function. The hippocampus develops during the first three postnatal weeks in rodents and is equivalent to the development of the human hippocampus that occurs during the third trimester (Clancy, Finlay, Darlington, & Anand, 2007; Clancy, Kersh et al., 2007; Winzer-Serhan, 2008). Therefore, if the focus of a study is to examine the long-term effects of MA exposure during hippocampal development on cognition later in life, we cannot model human *in utero* MA exposure by only exposing rodents to MA during gestation by injecting the pregnant mother with MA. Based on the pioneering work of Williams and Vorhees in rats (Vorhees et al., 2000; Vorhees, Skelton, & Williams, 2007; Williams et al., 2003), we have been using a neonatal MA exposure mouse model in which the mice are exposed to MA during the first three weeks of life to model human *in utero* MA exposure during hippocampal development. One advantage of this model is that it removes the potential effects of altered maternal care due to drug administration and withdrawal. Early life parental care can affect cognition later in life and postnatal exposure to MA controls for this possibility (Bredy, Lee, Meaney, & Brown, 2004; Rice, Sandman, Lenjavi, & Baram, 2008). Furthermore, postnatal exposure controls for potential variations in the dose of MA that each pup might receive *in utero* depending on the size of the litter.

Exposure to MA from postnatal days (PD) 11-20 causes hippocampus-dependent cognitive impairments in adolescence (Siegel, Park, & Raber, 2011) and adulthood (Acevedo, de Esch, & Raber, 2007; Siegel, Craytor, & Raber, 2010; Vorhees et al., 2000) in rodents. In general, female mice are more severely affected than male mice by the long-term effects of neonatal MA exposure on hippocampal function.

The Role of the Hippocampus in Cognition

The hippocampus is an area of the brain that is intimately involved in cognitive function. Lesions of the hippocampus in rodents cause deficits in working memory in the T-maze, spatial learning and memory in the water maze, and impair acquisition of passive avoidance (Deacon, Bannerman, Kirby, Croucher, & Rawlins, 2002; Gerlai, McNamara, Williams, & Phillips, 2002; Morris, Garrud, Rawlins, & O'Keefe, 1982). Hippocampal lesions in rats also impair contextual, but not cued, fear conditioning memory (Otto & Poon, 2006; R. G. Phillips & LeDoux, 1992) and impair novel location recognition and context memory, but not novel object recognition memory (Mumby, Gaskin, Glenn, Schramek, & Lehmann, 2002; Save, Poucet, Foreman, & Buhot, 1992).

The novel location recognition test is a spatial memory test, whereas the novel object recognition test does not have a spatial component. Thus the hippocampus is important for various forms of learning and memory that involve a spatial and contextual component and if the hippocampus is affected by neonatal MA exposure one would expect these cognitive functions to be affected. The water maze (Figure 1) and object recognition tests are particularly sensitive to detect effects of neonatal MA exposure on cognition later in life.

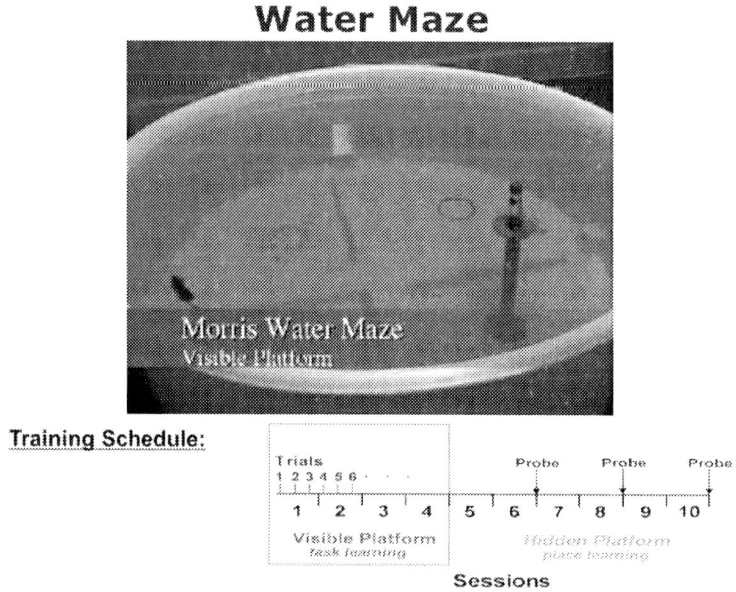

Figure 1. Water maze test. Mice are dropped at selected locations in a specific order and must locate the submerged platform on which a visible cue is placed. In later trials, the visible cue is removed, and the water is made opaque by a non-toxic, non-abrasive agent such as powdered milk or chalk to hide the platform. During hidden platform training, the target platform is removed to evaluate the spatial memory retention of the mouse in probe trials. A mouse with spatial memory retention preferentially searches the quadrant, which previously contained the platform (target quadrant). Data are recorded with a videotracking system (Noldus Instruments EthoVision), and later analyzed to calculate swim speeds, the time (latency) and distance moved to locate the platform, and the time spent in the target quadrant in relation to the other three quadrants during the probe trial.

Neurotransmitter Systems Implicated in the Effects of MA on the Brain

Most research has focused on MA exposure in the adult brain and the role of monoamine neurotransmitters, specifically dopamine (DA), serotonin (5-HT), and norepinephrine (NE), in the effects of MA on brain function (Katzung, 2007; Sulzer et al., 2005). MA acts as a substrate for the vesicular monoamine transporter. Once transported into the vesicle, MA binds free protons and alters the acidic pH of the vesicles, causing monoamine release into the cytosol (Sulzer et al., 2005). MA also acts at the plasma membrane transporters. It is unclear whether MA acts to block the uptake of monoamines from the synaptic cleft or if MA itself is a substrate for the transporters and induces reverse-transport of monoamines into the synaptic cleft (Sulzer et al., 2005). Regardless of the precise mechanism, MA increases non-vesicular release of DA, 5-HT, and NE and prevents their reuptake from the synaptic cleft (Katzung, 2007; Sulzer et al., 2005).

MA has long-term toxic effects on the adult brain. MA users who are abstinent for 3 months show reduced levels of the DA transporter (DAT) in the striatum and users who are abstinent up to 5 years show reduced levels of the 5-HT transporter (SERT) in the thalamus, caudate, putamen, and amygdala compared to non- users (Johanson et al., 2006; Sekine et al., 2006; Volkow et al., 2001). In adult rodents, SERT and DAT levels in the nucleus accumbens are reduced 2 weeks following MA exposure (Broening, Pu, & Vorhees, 1997; Guilarte, Nihei, McGlothan, & Howard, 2003). Immunoreactivity for tyrosine hydroxylase, the rate-limiting enzyme in the synthesis of DA, is reduced 60 days following MA exposure in adult rats in the nucleus accumbens, frontal cortex, and ventral tegmental area (VTA) (Trulson, Cannon, Faegg, & Raese, 1987). In addition, MA causes reductions in DA and 5-HT concentrations in the nucleus accumbens (Wallace, Gudelsky, & Vorhees, 1999), the number of 5-HT_2 receptors in the hippocampus, and DA D_1 and D_2 receptors in the nucleus accumbens and the caudate-putamen (McCabe, Hanson, Dawson, Wamsley, & Gibb, 1987). In this chapter we will review especially the role of the cholinergic and histaminergic systems in the long-term effects of MA exposure during brain development on brain function later in life. These two systems are relatively understudied in the context of MA exposure during brain development but play important roles in hippocampus-dependent learning and memory. Two previous studies have shown reduced acetylcholinesterase (AChE)-positive fibers in the cortex and dentate gyrus in adult male gerbils exposed to a single toxic dose of MA on PD 14 (Busche, Bagorda, Lehmann, Neddens, & Teuchert-Noodt, 2006; Lehmann, Hundsdorfer, Hartmann, & Teuchert-Noodt, 2004). Furthermore, as described in more detail below, two studies supported a role for the histaminergic system in the long-term effects of MA exposure during hippocampal development on cognition later in life (Acevedo et al., 2007; Acevedo, Pfankuch, van Meer, & Raber, 2008)

ROLE OF THE HISTAMINERGIC SYSTEM IN COGNITION

In the central nervous system (CNS), synthesis of L-histidine into histamine (HA) by L-histidine decarboxylase (HDC) takes place in a restricted population of neurons located in the tuberomammillary nucleus (TM) of the posterior hypothalamus. From the TM, histaminergic neurons project to virtually the entire brain, and, in the CNS, HA is involved in many important physiological processes, including the release of stress hormones such as corticotropin-releasing factor (CRF) and arginine vasopressin (AVP) (for a review, see Brown, Stevens, & Haas, 2001). Four distinct HA receptors, which are all G-protein-coupled receptors (GPCRs), have been identified. H_1 receptors, which couple to $G_{q/11}$ proteins, are expressed in the CNS, especially in the thalamus, hippocampus, cortex, amygdala, and in the basal forebrain (BF). Mobilization of calcium from intracellular Ca^{2+} stores is the main action of H_1 receptors. Besides increasing inositol phosphate accumulation that further increases Ca^{2+} flow, Ca^{2+} is, among other things, also responsible for the induction of nitric oxide production, leading to relaxation of the endothelium (Izumi, Makino, Shirakawa, & Garfield, 1995; Li et al., 2003). H_2 receptors, expressed in the periphery and in the CNS, couple to G_s proteins. In the CNS, the H_2 receptor is widely expressed with particularly high receptor density in the basal ganglia, the hippocampus and amygdala. High expression is also found in pyramidal cells of Ammon's horn, raphe nuclei, and the substantia nigra. In the CNS, H_2 receptor activation is associated with excitation through a blocking effect of Ca^{2+} and K^+ channels, regulation of fluid balance, and regulation of hormonal secretion. The H_3 receptor functions as an autoreceptor and enables HA to inhibit its own release (Arrang, Garbarg, & Schwartz, 1983; Bockaert & Pin, 1999; Lovenberg et al., 1999; Uveges et al., 2002). Thus, stimulation of H_3 receptors by H_3 agonists inhibits HA synthesis and release, while inhibition of H_3 receptors by H_3 receptor antagonists increases HA release (Arrang et al., 1983; Jansen, Mochizuki, Yamamoto, Timmerman, & Yamatodani, 1998). Endogenous release of HA in the brain is mainly regulated by H_3 receptors. In the CNS, high densities of H_3 receptors have been found in nucleus accumbens, striatum, olfactory tubercles, substantia nigra and the amygdala. Lower receptor densities have been detected in the hypothalamus. The H_3 receptor is a constitutively active receptor (Wieland et al., 2001) that mediates its effects through the $G_{i/o}$ class of G-proteins (Clark & Hill, 1996). In addition to HA, H_3 receptor-mediated signaling also affects other neurotransmitters such as DA (Schlicker, Fink, Detzner, & Gothert, 1993), 5-HT (Schlicker, Betz, & Gothert, 1988; Schlicker,

Schunack, & Gothert, 1990), GABA (Garcia, Floran, Arias-Montano, Young, & Aceves, 1997), NE (Silver et al., 2001), and various peptides (Hill et al., 1997). The H_4 receptor is not as widely expressed as other HA receptors (Nakamura, Itadani, Hidaka, Ohta, & Tanaka, 2000). In the CNS, H_4 receptors are mainly found in the cerebellum and at much lower levels in the hippocampus (Coge, Guenin, Rique, Boutin, & Galizzi, 2001).

The fetal rodent brain expresses H_1, H_2, and H_3 receptors (Karlstedt, Ahman, Anichtchik, Soinila, & Panula, 2003; Kinnunen, Lintunen, Karlstedt, Fukui, & Panula, 1998). At embryonic day (E) 15, HA is transiently produced in a subgroup of neurons in the raphe nucleus (Auvinen & Panula, 1988) and H_1, H_2, and H_3 receptors are expressed in the ventricular neuroepithelium in the midbrain and medulla (Karlstedt et al., 2003; Kinnunen et al., 1998). At E16, H_3 receptor mRNA is strongly expressed in thalamus, hypothalamus, midbrain, and cortex (Karlstedt et al., 2003), which are target areas for developing raphe neurons whose fibers contain HA (Vanhala, Yamatodani, & Panula, 1994) and later in development for HA neurons from the TM (Auvinen & Panula, 1988). At E19 and at birth, H_3 receptor mRNA is expressed in the cortical plate, cortical layer 6b, and nucleus accumbens (Karlstedt et al., 2003).

Studies with [^{3}H] mepyramine and [^{3}H] R*a*-methylhistamine have been performed to evaluate the postnatal developmental profile of H_1 and H_3 receptors, respectively. H_1 receptors are detected first at PD 2. In contrast, H_3 receptors are detected first at PD 9. H_1 receptors are detected at higher levels in the hypothalamus, hippocampus, and amygdala, while lower levels are detected in cortex, striatum, thalamus, and substantia nigra (Ryu, Yanai, Sakurai, Kim, & Watanabe, 1995). Resembling the changes in neuronal HA, H_1 receptor binding increases (without changes in affinity) from birth to adult levels at PD 25–30 (Subramanian, Whitmore, Seidler, & Slotkin, 1981; Tran, Freeman, Chang, & Snyder, 1980).

Most studies have focused on the short-term effects of HA receptor-mediated signaling on learning and memory. For example, in adulthood both positive and negative effects of neuronal HA on cognitive function have been reported. H_3 receptor stimulation improves memory retention in the water maze (Rubio, Begega, Santin, & Arias, 2002) and H_3 receptor blockade impairs social memory (Prast, Argyriou, & Philippu, 1996) and object recognition (Bongers, Leurs, Robertson, & Raber, 2004). Mice lacking H_1 receptors show less social isolation stress-induced impairments in cognition than wild-type mice (Dai et al., 2005). In addition, bilateral lesion of the TMs improves learning and memory in adult and aged animals (Huston, Wagner, & Hasenohrl, 1997).

In contrast to the results described above, H_3 receptor blockade might be beneficial under conditions of cognitive impairments caused by cholinergic dysfunction (Ghi, Orsetti, Gamalero, & Ferretti, 1999; Giovannini, Bartolini, Bacciottini, Greco, & Blandina, 1999; Miyazaki, Onodera, Imaizumi, & Timmerman, 1997). The link between HA and the cholinergic system might also be important in the context of long-term effects of neonatal MA exposure (see below).

In adulthood, there is a link between HA and MA. HA and its precursor L-histidine inhibit MA-induced stereotyped behavior and behavioral sensitization to MA, and these effects are blocked in the presence of H_1 or H_2 receptor antagonists (Ito, Onodera, Watanabe, & Sato, 1997). Similarly, behavioral sensitization to MA is also enhanced in mice lacking HDC (for a review, see Watanabe & Yanai, 2001). In contrast, in adult rodents, MA induces HA release in various brain regions and chronic MA administration increases cortical HA levels (Dai et al., 2004). In addition, H_3 receptor antagonists potentiate MA self-administration and MA- induced accumbal DA release (Munzar, Tanda, Justinova, & Goldberg, 2004), as well as the discriminative-stimulus effects of MA (Mori, Narita, Onodera, & Suzuki, 2002; Munzar, Nosal, & Goldberg, 1998). As described below, there is also a link between developmental MA exposure and HA.

The Role of the Histaminergic System in the Effects of MA Exposure during Brain Development on Cognition Later in Life

Adult female mice are more severely affected by neonatal MA exposure than adult male mice (Acevedo et al., 2007; Siegel et al., 2010), perhaps due to enhanced release of HA (Acevedo et al., 2007). Neonatal MA exposure increases HA levels in the brain compared to saline (SA) exposure (Acevedo et al., 2008). In addition, increasing HA release with the H_3 receptor antagonist thioperamide (THIO) from PD 11-20 mimics the detrimental effects of MA on cognition at 3 months of age (Acevedo et al., 2007). Neonatal exposure to MA and THIO might also have similar effects on cognition during adolescence. Therefore, we assessed behavioral performance in adolescent mice following neonatal exposure to MA or THIO.

Eleven total litters of C57BL/6J mouse pups were bred in our colony using breeding cages containing one male and two female adult mice. Female mice were singly housed from the first sign of pregnancy. Litter sizes of 2–10 pups were injected using a within-litter design to balance the number of distinct treatment injections within a litter and across sexes. Every litter contained up to 4 MA-injected pups. Lab chow (PicoLab Rodent Diet 20, #5053; PMI Nutrition International, St. Louis, MO) and water were given *ad libitum*. (*d*)-MA hydrocholoride (5 mg/kg), obtained from the Research Triangle Institute (Research Triangle Park, NC) through the National Institute on Drug Abuse drug supply program, or the histamine H_3 receptor antagonist THIO (5 mg/kg) synthesized by Dr. de Esch (Free University, Amterdam, The Netherlands), were diluted with 0.9% sodium chloride (SA) to the appropriate concentration. These MA and THIO doses produce activation of the hypothalamic-pituitary-adrenal axis in PD 11-20 mice (Acevedo et al., 2008) as well as cognitive impairments and reduced levels of the dendritic marker microtubule-associated protein 2 (MAP-2) immunoreactivity in the hippocampus and cortex of PD 90 mice (Acevedo et al., 2007; Acevedo et al., 2008; Siegel et al., 2010). Male and female pups were weighed and injected with MA, THIO, or SA from PD 11-20 (injection volume of 0.1 mL), once daily between 6:30 and 9:00 AM. On PD 21, pups were weaned and group housed with five mice per cage according to sex. The litters were provided with soft foods to maintain stable weight gain. The mice were kept on a 12 hour light/dark schedule (lights on at 06:00). Behavioral testing took place during the light cycle. All procedures conformed to the standards of the National Institutes of Health Guide for the Care and Use of Laboratory Animals and were approved by the Animal Care and Use Committee of the Oregon Health and Science University.

Beginning on PD 28, mice were individually housed. Behavioral testing began on PD 30. The water maze was used to assess spatial learning and memory requiring navigation. The mice were first trained to locate four visible platform locations (Sessions 1-4) and subsequently, trained to locate two hidden platform locations (Sessions 5-8 and 9-12, respectively). Probe trial tests (no platform) were used to assess whether mice showed a bias towards the learned hidden platform location. A circular pool (140 cm diameter) was filled with water made opaque by adding chalk (22° C $\pm$ 2° C) and contained a platform (20 cm wide) approximately 1 cm below water level. On the first two days of water maze testing, mice were first trained to locate a visible platform (platform flagged with a visible beacon) in two trials per session with five-minute inter-trial intervals and two sessions per day (two hours apart). Trials ended when mice reached the platform and remained on it for 10 seconds or when 60 seconds elapsed, at which point the mice were guided to the platform and allowed to remain on it for 10 seconds. Swim speeds during visible platform training were used to assess potential differences in vision, locomotion, motivation, and differences in task learning. After visible platform training, the mice were trained to locate a hidden platform in two trials per session with five-minute inter-trial intervals and two sessions per day (two hours apart). On days 3 and 4, the location of the hidden platform remained constant while the drop location varied for each trial. On days 5 and 6, the platform was moved to a new location (reversal training) and the mice were trained to locate the novel platform location using the same number of trials and sessions used for the first platform location. A 60 second probe trial test (platform removed) was conducted 1 hour after the last trial of the fourth and sixth day of hidden platform training. Performance measures for visible and hidden platform location training included swim speeds, time to reach the platform (latency), and total distance swam. For the probe trials, spatial memory retention (target preference or bias) was assessed by analyzing how much time the mice spent in the quadrant where the platform was located during hidden training (target quadrant) versus the three non-target quadrants. In addition, the percent of mice within each treatment group that showed a spatial bias and spent more time in the target quadrant than any other quadrant was analyzed. The swimming patterns of the mice were analyzed using the EthoVision video tracking system set at 6 samples/second.

For the water maze platform training trials, data were analyzed using repeated measures analysis of variance (ANOVA) with sex and treatment as between subject-factors and session as the within subject factor. Visible and hidden platform training sessions were analyzed separately. Violations of Maulchy's Test of Sphericity in the repeated measures ANOVAs were addressed using the Greenhouse-Geisser correction. For the water maze probe trial analysis of target preference, one-way ANOVAs were used to assess the effect of quadrant within each group. Where appropriate within each group, Tukey's post-hoc tests were used to compare time in the target quadrant versus time in the three non-target quadrants.

The latency to the platform was used as a measure of performance since there were no group differences in swim speeds during the visible platform training sessions. All groups of mice learned the task and improved their performance during the visible platform training (effect of session: F (1.96, 82.47) = 56.46; $p < 0.001$). There were no significant effects of the treatments, sex, or interactions between them (data not shown). During the hidden platform training sessions, all groups of mice learned the first (F (2.51, 105.34) = 10.89; $p < 0.001$) and second (F (3, 126) = 29.45; $p < 0.001$) platform location. There were no significant effects of the treatments, sex, or interactions between them (data not shown). Similar data were obtained when total distance swam was analyzed as the performance measure. However, group differences were seen when spatial memory retention was assessed in the probe trials. Following hidden platform training for the first platform location, SA-treated female mice showed spatial memory retention but MA-treated female did not (Figure 2). No detrimental effects were seen in THIO-treated female or THIO- or MA-treated male mice. These data show that neonatal MA exposure causes sex-dependent impairments in spatial memory retention. In the second probe trial, following reversal training, SA- and MA-treated female mice showed spatial memory retention but THIO-treated female mice did not (data not shown).

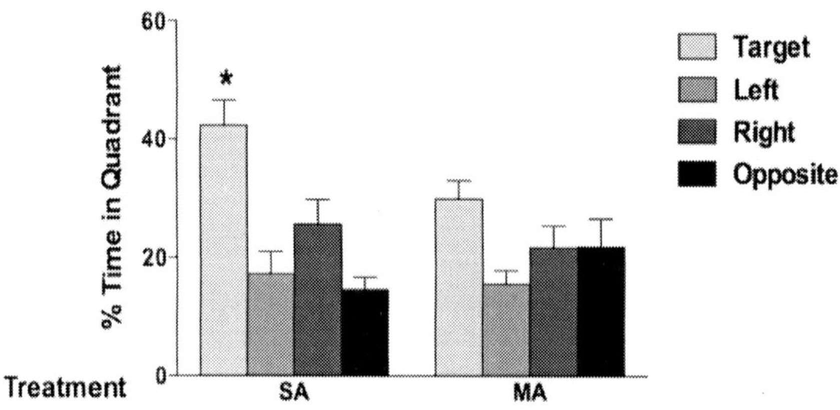

Figure 2. Neonatal female mice treated with MA (5 mg/kg) or SA from PD 11-20 were behaviorally tested starting on PD 30. The mice were trained to locate a visible platform on days 1 and 2 and a hidden platform on days 3 and 4. One hour after the last training trial on day 4, spatial memory retention was assessed in a probe trial (no platform). While SA-treated female mice searched most time in the target quadrant that contained the platform previously, MA-treated female mice did not. $N = 8$ mice/treatment. *$p < 0.05$ versus any other quadrant.

The percentage of mice in each group spending more time in the target quadrant than any other quadrant was also analyzed. Among the female mice in the first probe trial, less than 50% of the MA-treated mice showed a spatial bias (37%) while the majority of SA-treated (62.5%) and THIO-treated (87.5%) mice did. In the second probe trial, while the majority of SA- and

MA-treated mice showed spatial bias (SA: 71% and MA: 100%), the majority of THIO-treated mice did not (50%). These data show that compared to neonatal SA exposure, neonatal MA exposure causes impairments in hippocampus-dependent spatial memory retention while neonatal THIO exposure causes-subtle impairments in spatial memory retention in a reversal task among adolescent female mice. Such effects were not seen in the male mice. Similar results were seen in adult mice following neonatal MA exposure (Acevedo et al., 2007). While MA-treated female mice did not show spatial memory retention, MA-treated male mice did. In contrast to MA, THIO-treated adolescent and adult female mice did not show impairments in spatial memory retention in the first probe trial. However, when adolescent mice were trained to locate a second platform location during reversal training, THIO-treated female mice did show impairments in spatial memory retention. It is possible that a higher dose of THIO might also cause impairments in spatial memory retention in the first probe trial.

In contrast to the water maze, no sex-dependent effects of neonatal MA exposure were found in hippocampus-dependent novel location recognition in adolescence mice (Siegel, Park et al., 2011) while such sex-dependent effects on novel location recognition were seen in adulthood (Acevedo et al., 2007; Siegel et al., 2010). Table 1 summarizes the cognitive data of adolescent and adult mice following neonatal MA exposure. As both the first water maze probe trial and novel location recognition are hippocampus-dependent tasks, these data show that the water maze is particularly sensitive to detect sex-dependent effects of neonatal MA exposure on spatial memory retention and that neonatal MA exposure impairs performance on these hippocampus-dependent cognitive tests. Based on the link between HA and the cholinergic system, alterations in the cholinergic system might mediate the effects of altered HA levels following neonatal MA exposure.

Table 1. Summary of novel location recognition and spatial memory retention of mice exposed to MA during hippocampal development

Age group	Novel location recognition	Spatial memory retention (water maze)
Cognition in adolescence	Impaired in female and male mice	Impaired in female, but not male, mice
Cognition in adulthood	Impaired in female, but not male, mice	Impaired in female, but not male, mice

Role of the Cholinergic System in Cognition

The BF is one of the most prominent cholinergic nuclei in the brain and contains four separate groups of cholinergic neurons: the medial septum (MS), vertical limb nucleus of the diagonal band (VDB), horizontal limb nucleus of the diagonal band (HDB), and the nucleus basalis of Meynert (NB) (Feldman, Meyer, & Quenzer, 1997; Halbach & Dermietzel, 2002; Mesulam, Mufson, Wainer, & Levey, 1983). The MS and VDB neurons are the major source of cholinergic innervation in the hippocampus (Gaykema, Luiten, Nyakas, & Traber, 1990; Linke, Schwegler, & Boldyreva, 1994), while the cholinergic neurons in the NB project mainly to the amygdala and cortex (Gaykema et al., 1990; Halbach & Dermietzel, 2002; Houser, Crawford, Barber, Salvaterra, & Vaughn, 1983; Mesulam et al., 1983; Zaborszky, Carlsen, Brashear, & Heimer, 1986). There are two classes of acetylcholine (ACh) receptors: nicotinic ACh receptors (nAChRs) and muscarinic ACh receptors (mAChRs) (Cummings, 2000; Feldman et al., 1997; Halbach & Dermietzel, 2002). The nAChRs are ligand-gated ion channels comprised of five membrane-spanning subunits in a 2α3β subunit or 5α7 subunit stoichiometry (Halbach & Dermietzel, 2002; Paterson & Nordberg, 2000). In the CNS, the nAChRs are located on both pre- and post-synaptic membranes (Halbach & Dermietzel, 2002; Paterson & Nordberg, 2000). Ligand binding studies and *in vivo* imaging studies in humans reveal that nAChRs are expressed primarily in the cortex, thalamus, hippocampus, striatum, cerebellum, and BF (Paterson & Nordberg, 2000). The α7 nAChRs show highest expression levels in the hippocampus (Paterson & Nordberg, 2000). The mAChRs are metabotropic GPCRs. There are five mAChRs subtypes: M_1, M_3, and M_5 mAChRs (M_1-type) and M_2 and M_4 mAChRs (M_2-type). The M_1-type mAChRs are coupled to the $G_{q/11}$ protein, which increases neuronal excitation while the M_2-type mAChRs are coupled to the $G_{i/o}$ protein, which reduces neuronal excitation. The M_2-type receptors are often located on the pre-synaptic terminals of cholinergic neurons and provide negative feedback on ACh release. The mAChRs are more widely distributed throughout the mammalian brain compared to the nAChRs. The M_1 mAChRs are most commonly expressed in the cortex, hippocampus, amygdala, striatum, and olfactory bulb while the M_2 mAChRs are located in areas of the brain containing cholinergic neurons such as the BF and the pontomesencephalic nuclei, but are also found in the thalamus, hippocampus, cortex, brainstem, striatum, and cerebellum. The M_3 mAChRs are found primarily in the cortex, olfactory bulb, striatum, thalamus, and brain stem. The distribution of the M_4 mAChRs is similar to that of the M_1

mAChRs, except levels are higher in the striatum. Finally the M_5 mAChRs show very low levels in most areas of the mammalian brain (Aubert, Cecyre, Gauthier, & Quirion, 1992; Halbach & Dermietzel, 2002; Schwab, Bruckner, Rothe, Castellano, & Oliverio, 1992).

During development, BF ACh neurons migrate prenatally but continue to develop mature phenotypes well into postnatal development. In C57BL/6J mice, mitotically-active cells in the germinal zone of the lateral ventricle are present from E12-17. These cells divide in the germinal zone and migrate to their final destination in the BF prior to birth (Brady, Phelps, & Vaughn, 1989; Schambra, Sulik, Petrusz, & Lauder, 1989). Choline acetyltransferase (ChAT), the enzyme that synthesizes ACh, shows low activity during gestation in rodents. However, activity levels increase substantially after birth, peaking around PD 30 in rats in the BF. A similar developmental pattern occurs for AChE activity in the BF (Thal, Gilbertson, Armstrong, & Gage, 1992). In the hippocampus, AChE and ChAT activity levels are nearly undetectable during gestation and show large increases from birth until PD 30 in rats (Thal et al., 1992). Similarly, peak AChE and ChAT activity levels are reached in the frontal cortex of rats on approximately PD 30 (Thal et al., 1992; Zahalka, Seidler, Lappi, Yanai, & Slotkin, 1993).

The ACh receptor subtypes show differential developmental timelines, with the nAChRs developing prenatally and the mAChRs developing postnatally in rodents. The α7 nAChRs appear in the hippocampus as early as E12 in rats (Abreu-Villaca, Filgueiras, & Manhaes, 2010). Similar early development of nAChRs has been shown in humans, with mRNA for various subunits seen in fetuses as early as week 5 of gestation. Cortical mRNA levels are detected beginning at gestational week 6 (Hellstrom-Lindahl, Gorbounova, Seiger, Mousavi, & Nordberg, 1998). Binding studies in humans substantiate these findings, with α4β2 nAChR binding increasing from gestational week 4-12 (Hellstrom-Lindahl et al., 1998). In contrast, M_1 mAChRs levels are very low prior to birth and show large increases after birth and up to PD 21 and 35 in the rat hippocampus and cortex, respectively (Aubert, Cecyre, Gauthier, & Quirion, 1996). The M_2 mAChRs show large increases in receptor binding sites between PD 20-40 in cortical regions and maximal levels on PD 21 in the hippocampus of the rat (Aubert et al., 1996). A similar late pattern of mAChR development is observed in humans. The mAChRs appear around weeks 16-18 of gestation and represent approximately 24% of the receptor density at birth in the frontal cortex. Between weeks 24-32 there is a dramatic increase in mAChR binding sites, with over 60% of the total receptors found at birth developing during the third trimester (Ravikumar & Sastry, 1985).

The cholinergic system plays an important role in cognition. For example, cortical ACh release increases during performance of attention-demanding tasks (Arnold, Burk, Hodgson, Sarter, & Bruno, 2002; Dalley et al., 2001; Himmelheber, Sarter, & Bruno, 2000; Passetti, Dalley, O'Connell, Everitt, & Robbins, 2000) and hippocampal ACh release increases during memory retrieval in contextual fear conditioning tests in rats (Nail-Boucherie, Dourmap, Jaffard, & Costentin, 2000). Lesions of the BF in rats impair target detection (Risbrough, Bontempi, & Menzaghi, 2002) and response accuracy (Muir, Everitt, & Robbins, 1994) in the 5-choice serial reaction time task (5-SRTT), an attention test for rodents (Robbins, 2002). AChE inhibitors improve attentional performance on the 5-SRTT in BF-lesioned rats and enhance object location memory in mice (Muir et al., 1994; Murai, Okuda, Tanaka, & Ohta, 2007). Similar impairments in attention following BF lesions are seen in non-human primates (Voytko et al., 1994). Specific lesions of the cholinergic BF neurons in rats impair spatial learning and memory in the water maze (Frick, Kim, & Baxter, 2004; Lin, LeBlanc, Deacon, & Isacson, 1998).

Studies in both rodents and primates demonstrate the importance of the ACh receptors in cognition. The nAChRs play an important role in cognitive function (for a review, see Paterson & Nordberg, 2000). Nicotine, a potent nAChR agonist, improves learning and memory in a spatial discrimination task in rats with septum lesions (Decker, Majchrzak, & Anderson, 1992) and improves attention in rodents (J. M. Phillips, McAlonan, Robb, & Brown, 2000; Young et al., 2004). Mice lacking the α7 nAChR show impairments in the 5-SRTT and olfactory working memory span performance (Young et al., 2007). In humans, acute nicotine administration decreases reaction time and increases target detection accuracy and memory recognition (Froeliger, Gilbert, & McClernon, 2009).

Blockade of the mAChRs in rodents impairs spatial learning in the water maze (Fontana, Inouye, & Johnson, 1994), passive avoidance retention memory (Fontana et al., 1994), object location recognition memory (Murai et al., 2007), memory in a delayed non-matching to position task (van Hest, Stroet, van Haaren, & Feenstra, 1990), spatial discrimination learning (Steckler & Holsboer, 2001), contextual and cued fear memory (Feiro & Gould, 2005; Rogers & Kesner, 2004), sensorimotor gating in the pre-pulse inhibition (PPI) test (Jones & Shannon, 2000), and attention in the 5-SRTT (Mirza & Stolerman, 2000; Ruotsalainen, Miettinen, MacDonald, Koivisto, & Sirvio, 2000). mAChR blockade also impairs object recognition memory in adult rats, an effect that is reversed by AChE inhibitors and nicotine (Sambeth, Riedel, Smits, & Blokland, 2007). Scopolamine, a general mAChR antagonist, impairs object recognition and the number of words recalled in a working memory task while AChE inhibitors improve reaction time on a working memory task in humans (Thiel, 2003). Thus, the cholinergic system is important in a variety of cognitive tasks in multiple species.

Cholinergic disruption during brain development induces cognitive impairments later in life (for a review, see Berger-Sweeney, 2003). Irreversible cholinergic BF lesions on PD 7 impair memory for social olfactory information (Ricceri et al., 2004) and spatial learning in the water maze (Pappas, Payne, Fortin, & Sherren, 2005) in male rats in adulthood. Cholinergic BF lesions on PD 1 or 3 impair acquisition of a passive avoidance task in adolescent female rats and impair novel location recognition memory in adult male and female rats (Ricceri, Hohmann, & Berger-Sweeney, 2002). Irreversible lesions of the NB on PD 1 reduce spatial learning in the water maze in male mice at 8 weeks of age (Arters, Hohmann, Mills, Olaghere, & Berger-Sweeney, 1998).

Effects of MA Exposure during Hippocampal Development on the Cholinergic System Later in Life

Very little is known about the long-term effects of developmental MA exposure on the cholinergic system. The majority of the literature on MA and ACh focuses on the adult brain and will be briefly described prior to discussing the effects of MA exposure during brain development. Heavy MA use reduces the activity of ChAT in various areas of the adult human brain, including the caudate and the hippocampus (Kish et al., 1999; Siegal et al., 2004). Heavy MA use in adult humans is also associated with a 48% increase in concentrations of the vesicular ACh transporter in the caudate (Siegal et al., 2004). High doses of MA acutely increase ACh levels in the VTA (Dobbs & Mark, 2008), interpeduncular nucleus (Hussain, Taraschenko, & Glick, 2008), and the striatum (Taguchi et al., 1998) in adult rodents and reduce the total number of cholinergic cells in the dorsal striatum of adult rats (Zhu, Xu, & Angulo, 2006). Additionally, MA alters both types of ACh receptors: the nAChRs up-regulate in cell culture following MA incubation (Garcia-Rates, Camarasa, Escubedo, & Pubill, 2007) while the mAChRs down-regulate in the striatum, cortex, and hippocampus following MA exposure in adult rats (McCabe, Gibb, Wamsley, & Hanson, 1987).

Animal models of MA exposure during brain development have typically focused on the long-term effects of MA in adulthood whereas relatively little research has focused on the effects in adolescence. Furthermore, no studies have examined the effects of MA exposure during brain development on the adolescent cholinergic system. Therefore, in this chapter we will focus on the effects of neonatal MA exposure on the BF cholinergic system seen in adolescence.

ChAT is commonly used as marker for cholinergic cells and processes (Oda, 1999). To determine the effects of neonatal MA exposure on the BF cholinergic system, we analyzed ChAT expression in the BF, hippocampus, and cortex. The mAChRs are present in high concentrations in these brain regions (Aubert et al., 1992; Halbach & Dermietzel, 2002; Paterson & Nordberg, 2000). Therefore, mAChR binding was also examined in the hippocampus and cortex. The BF also contains non-cholinergic neurons that are GABAergic or glutamatergic and play an important role in BF signaling and function (Gritti, Mainville, & Jones, 1993, 1994; Gritti, Manns, Mainville, & Jones, 2003; Henny & Jones, 2006; Manns, Mainville, & Jones, 2001; Mesulam, 2004). GABAergic BF neurons project along with cholinergic neurons to the hippocampus and the cortex (Freund & Antal, 1988; Freund & Meskenaite, 1992; Linke et al., 1994). Parvalbumin (PVA) is a calcium-binding protein that is expressed in many GABAergic cells and is commonly used as a GABAergic marker in the mammalian brain. PVA-positive cells in the BF do not express ChAT (Gritti et al., 1993; Kiss, Patel, Baimbridge, & Freund, 1990) and nearly all PVA-positive BF cells also stain positive for GABAergic markers (Freund, 1989; Gritti et al., 2003). Therefore, the BF GABAergic neurons were also assessed following MA exposure using PVA.

Three- to 5-month-old male and female C57BL/6J mice were bred in our colony using breeding cages containing one male and two female mice. Female mice were singly housed from the first sign of pregnancy. Lab chow (PicoLab Rodent Diet 20, #5053; PMI Nutrition International, St. Louis, MO) and water were given *ad libitum*. (*d*)-MA hydrochloride (5 mg/kg), obtained from the Research Triangle Institute (Research Triangle Park, NC) through the National Institute on Drug Abuse drug supply program, was diluted with 0.9% sodium chloride (SA) to the appropriate concentration. This dose of MA was selected based on previous findings that it causes long-term cognitive impairments in adolescent and adult mice exposed during postnatal hippocampal development (Acevedo et al., 2007; Siegel et al., 2010; Siegel, Park et al., 2011). Male and female pups from a total of 18 separate litters were weighed and given a single intra-peritoneal injection of MA or SA daily at 10:00 from PD 11-20 (injection volume of 0.1 mL). A within-litter injection design was used to balance the number of MA and SA injections within a litter and across sexes. On PD 21, pups were weaned and group housed with five mice per cage according to sex. Litters were provided soft foods during the injection period and two weeks after weaning to maintain stable weight gain. The mice were kept on a 12 hour light/dark schedule (lights on at 06:00). All procedures conformed to the standards of the National Institutes of Health Guide for the Care and Use of Laboratory Animals and were approved by the Animal Care and Use Committee of the Oregon Health and Science University.

On PD 30, mice were deeply anesthetized with a cocktail containing 100 mg/kg ketamine, 10 mg/kg xylazine, and 2 mg/kg acepromazine and were transcardially perfused with phosphate-buffered SA (PBS) followed by 4% paraformaldehyde (pH = 7.4). Brains were removed and post-fixed overnight in 4% paraformaldehyde at 4° C, transferred to 30% sucrose solution, and were embedded in cryoprotectant and stored at -80° C until sectioning. Serial coronal sections (50 μm) were collected onto Superfrost microscope slides (Fisher Scientific, Pittsburgh, PA) through the entire MS/VDB/HDB (MA: n = 10, SA: n = 10), NB (MA: n = 11, SA: n = 11) or hippocampus/cortex (MA: n = 10, SA: n = 9) with a 200 μm inter-section distance, guided by the mouse brain atlas (Franklin & Paxinos, 1997). Due to a lack of clear anatomical boundaries between the MS, VDB, and HDB, the MS/VDB/HDB was considered as one region and examined separately from the NB. For the MS/VDB/HDB region, a total of 6 sections were collected per mouse (+1.18 to 0.00 mm Bregma). For the NB, a total of 4 sections were collected per mouse (-0.25 to -1.00 mm Bregma). For the hippocampus/cortex, a total of 12 sections were collected per mouse (-1.00 mm to -4.00 mm Bregma). Sections were stained for immunoreactivity of ChAT. Following an antigen retrieval step according to the manufacturer's instructions (H-3000; Vector Laboratories, Burlingame, CA), sections were incubated for 2 hours at room temperature in a blocking solution (5% normal donkey serum in PBS containing 0.2% Triton X-100 and 0.2% bovine serum albumen (PBT)), followed by incubation overnight at 4° C in goat-anti-ChAT primary antibody (1:400; Millipore, Billerica, MA). Following 4 washes with PBT (10 min each) and 1 wash with PBS (15 min), sections were incubated for 2 hours at room temperature in donkey-anti-goat IgG antibody (1:50) conjugated to Texas Red for fluorescent visualization (Jackson Immunoresearch, West Grove, PA). Following 4 washes with PBT (10 min each) and 1 wash with PBS (15 min), the sections were covered with anti-fade solution containing a

DAPI counterstain (Vectashield, Vector Laboratories) and were coverslipped (Fisher Scientific). Slides were stored in the dark at 4° C until they were imaged.

NeuN is a marker of mature neurons and was used to quantify the total density of neurons in the BF (Mullen, Buck, & Smith, 1992). Procedures for PVA and NeuN immunohistochemistry were identical to those for ChAT, except that PVA and NeuN imaging were performed only on sections from the MS/VDB/HDB. The same PD 30 mice that were used for the ChAT-positive cell counts in the MS/VDB/HDVB were used for the current studies (MA: n = 10, SA: n = 10) and the sections were directly adjacent to those used for the ChAT-positive cell counts in the MS/VDB/HDB. Sections were stained for fluorescent visualization of PVA and NeuN. Following an antigen retrieval step according to the manufacturer's instructions (H-3000; Vector Laboratories), sections were incubated for 2 hours at room temperature in a blocking solution (5% normal donkey serum in PBS containing 0.05% Tween-20 (PT)), followed by incubation overnight at 4° C with guinea pig-anti-PVA (1:300; Chemicon International, Billerica, MA) and mouse-anti-NeuN (1:400; Millipore, Billerica, MA) primary antibodies. Following 4 washes with PT (10 min each) and 1 wash with PBS (15 min), sections were incubated with donkey-anti- guinea pig and donkey-anti-mouse IgG antibody (1:50 for each) conjugated to fluorescein isothiocyanate (PVA) or Texas Red (NeuN) for fluorescent visualization (Jackson Immunoresearch) for 2 hours at room temperature. Following 4 washes with PT (10 min each) and 1 wash with PBS (15 min), the sections were covered with anti-fade solution containing a DAPI counterstain (Vectashield, Vector Laboratories) and were coverslipped (Fisher Scientific). Slides were stored in the dark at 4° C until they were imaged.

The density of ChAT-positive cells in the MS/VDB/HDB and NB was calculated by counting the total number of cells found within the region, using an unbiased rare event stereological procedure. Because there are so few ChAT-positive cells in the BF, each cell was counted within the defined region in 6 separate sections for the MS/VDB/HDB and 4 separate sections for the NB using the 60X objective lens (N.A. = 1.42, W.D. = 0.15, F.N. = 26.5) of an Olympus spinning disc confocal microscope (IX81, Olympus Imaging Corp., Center Valley, PA) equipped with Slidebook software (Intelligent Imaging Solutions). The density of ChAT-positive cells within each section was calculated by dividing the number of counted cells by the sample volume. The average density was calculated by averaging the sample densities for each mouse.

The density of PVA-positive and NeuN-positive cells in the MS/VDB/HDB was estimated using the nonbiased stereological physical volume fractionator technique (West, Slomianka, & Gundersen, 1991) using the 60X objective lens of the confocal microscope equipped with Slidebook software. Six separate sections spanning the MS/VDB/HDB were imaged for each mouse using 15 separate dissectors for each section. Each dissector (50 x 50 μm) consisted of a stack of 10 images with a 2 μm inter-image distance. PVA-positive cells and NeuN-positive cells were counted when they appeared within the dissector in one image of the 10 image stack but not in the preceding image. Cells were counted only when the staining appeared with a distinctly labeled DAPI stained nucleus. Thus a total of approximately 90 individual dissectors were counted to obtain an unbiased and accurate average density of PVA-positive and NeuN-positive cells per cubic centimeter within the MS/VDB/HDB of each mouse. The density of PVA-positive and NeuN-positive cells within each dissector was averaged for each mouse across all sections.

Densitometry analysis was used to quantify the area occupied by ChAT-immunoreactive fibers innervating the hippocampus and cortex. Immunofluorescence was imaged in stacks of 10 images with a 1 μm inter-image range in selected sub-regions of the hippocampus (CA1, CA3, stratum radiatum of the CA1 and CA3, and the granule and molecular layer of the dentate gyrus) and cortex (motor, primary and secondary sensory, entorhinal and lateral entorhinal, and piriform cortex) using the 60X objective lens of a confocal microscope equipped with Slidebook software. Stacks of images were vertically collapsed into a single image using a summation algorithm. An intensity threshold was chosen for each group of brains stained together, containing mice from each treatment group, based on the average intensities of immunoreactivity. The total number of pixels with ChAT immunofluorescence intensity above the threshold was determined within each image and converted to area. Twelve sections per mouse were used.

A two-way ANOVA was used to assess the effects of treatment and sex on the density of ChAT-positive cells in the MS/VDB/HDB and NB, and the density of PVA-positive and NeuN-positive cells in the MS/VDB/HDB. A repeated measure ANOVA was used to assess the effects of treatment and sex on the area occupied by ChAT immunoreactivity in all regions of the hippocampus and cortex. Lower-bound estimates of epsilon were used for all repeated measures ANOVAs.

The volumes of the MS/VDB/HDB and the NB did not differ between MA- and SA-exposed or male and female mice (data not shown). For the density of ChAT-positive cells in the MS/VDB/HDB, there was an interaction between treatment and sex (F (1, 16) = 6.53, p = 0.02). Thus the effects of treatment were explored in male and female mice separately. There was no difference between MA- and SA-exposed males in the density of ChAT-positive cells. However, female MA-exposed mice had a higher density of ChAT-positive cells than female SA-exposed mice in the MS/VDB/HDB (F (1, 8) = 5.80, p = 0.04; Table 2). There was no effect of treatment on the density of ChAT-positive cells in the NB. Male mice, however, had a higher density of ChAT-positive cells in the NB compared to female mice (F (1, 18) = 8.15, p = 0.01; Table 2).

MA exposure during brain development did not alter the density of PVA-positive or NeuN-positive cells in the MS/VDB/HDB (Table 2). There was no difference between the treatment groups or sexes in the proportion of the percent of ChAT- positive (cholinergic), PVA-positive (GABAergic), or other neurons in the MS/VDB/HDB. However, in female mice, MA exposure significantly increased the percent of ChAT-positive cells compared to SA exposure (t (1, 20) = -2.17, p = 0.04; data not shown). Negative controls with secondary antibody only revealed no fluorescent visualization, indicating that all of the antibodies used were specific.

Table 2. Summary of the density of cholinergic, GABAergic, and total neurons in the basal forebrain in adolescent mice

Treat-ment	Sex	Cholinergic (MS/VDB/HDB)	Choli-nergic (NB)	GABA-ergic	Total Neurons
SA	Males	241.7 ± 47.6	144.8 ± 7.7[a]	57,868.7 ± 7048.2	101,147.9 ± 8803.9
MA	Males	142.0 ± 54.8	99.7 ± 18.5[a]	58,168.6 ± 11,803.2	91,057.7 ± 9848.3
SA	Femal es	146.5 ± 38.6	66.9 ± 6.8	57,742.2 ± 6960.4	96,231.1 ± 4371.1
MA	Femal es	280.5 ± 40.1*	87.3 ± 22.4	75,857.4 ± 12,690.5	97,402.5 ± 6985.3

Note: GABAergic (PVA-positive) cells and neurons (NeuN-positive) were examined only in the MS/VDB/HDB. Cholinergic cells (ChAT-positive) were examined in both the MS/VDB/HDB and the NB.

* MA-exposed female mice higher than SA-exposed female mice, $p < 0.05$.

[a] Male mice higher than female mice, $p < 0.05$ main effect of sex.

For the area occupied by ChAT-positive axons in the hippocampus, there was a treatment x sex interaction (F (1, 15) = 7.53, p = 0.02). The effects of treatment on the area occupied by ChAT immunoreactivity in all areas of the hippocampus collapsed together were explored in each sex separately as there was no interaction between treatment, sex, and region. In the male mice, there was no effect of treatment on the area occupied by ChAT-positive fibers. In contrast, female MA-exposed mice had a higher area occupied by ChAT-positive fibers in all regions of the hippocampus compared to female SA-exposed mice (F (1, 7) = 6.99, p = 0.03; Table 3). Unlike the hippocampus, there was no effect of treatment or sex on the area occupied by ChAT-positive fibers in the cortex (Table 3).

Table 3. Summary of the area occupied by cholinergic axons in the hippocampus and cortex in adolescent mice

Hippocampus Treatment	Sex	CA1	CA1SR	CA3	CA3SR	DGG	DGM
SA	Males	4497.6 ± 1025.9	4250.4 ± 644.8	5131.1 ± 1047.4	4925.6 ± 868.1	3274.8 ± 911.5	4605.5 ± 729.7
MA	Males	3108.8 ± 1072.0	3008.0 ± 1133.0	3649.3 ± 1211.4	3767.3 ± 1185.0	2335.5 ± 1040.0	2950.7 ± 1043.8
SA	Females	4468.3 ± 1554.8	5129.8 ± 1670.3	5468.9 ± 1698.9	5845.4 ± 1409.0	4187.9 ± 1492.2	5211.1 ± 1583.0
MA	Females	9643.9 ± 1187.8*	9992.9 ± 1207.2*	10,170.3 ± 874.5*	10,180.8 ± 851.2*	8260.1 ± 880.2*	9402.3 ± 903.4*
Cortex Treatment	Sex	Ent	Lateral Ent	Motor	Piriform	1° Sen	2° Sen
SA	Males	3487.7 ± 1202.3	2552.7 ± 622.4	2985.0 ± 596.7	3121.4 ± 732.3	2788.6 ± 947.7	2783.0 ± 1101.5
MA	Males	2377.5 ± 819.5	2449.8 ± 817.2	2518.5 ± 1790.9	3819.5 ± 928.0	2929.6 ± 1279.1	3298.8 ± 1226.1
SA	Females	3490.9 ± 957.2	4397.5 ± 1112.7	4789.3 ± 1717.4	3053.1 ± 795.8	4038.9 ± 1451.8	4212.7 ± 1896.8
MA	Females	4866.9 ± 954.9	5823.8 ± 1198.7	5346.7 ± 1688.6	5659.0 ± 1268.9	5666.8 ± 902.0	4221.7 ± 2096.1

Note: SR = stratum radiatum, DGG = dentate gyrus granule layer, DGM = dentate gyrus molecular layer, Ent = entorhinal, 1° Sen = primary sensory, 2° Sen = secondary sensory.

* MA-exposed female mice higher than SA-exposed female mice, $p < 0.05$.

Next, muscarinic receptor binding was assessed. Mice were killed by cervical dislocation on PD 30 and receptor saturation binding experiments were performed using hippocampal (MA: $n = 20$, SA: $n = 20$) and cortical (MA: $n = 13$, SA: $n = 14$) membrane preparations and radioligands specific for M_1 ([^{3}H] Pirenzepine) or M_2 ([^{3}H] AF-DX-384) mAChRs (Siegel, Benice, Van Meer, Park, & Raber, 2011; Vaucher et al., 2002; Watson, Roeske, & Yamamura, 1986). Bilateral hippocampi and cortices were dissected and freshly frozen. Tissue preparations were homogenized in 1 mL of ice-cold buffer (140 mmol NaCl, 0.2 mmol KCl, 10 mmol $MgCl_2$, 0.5 mmol EDTA, 50 mmol Tris, pH = 7.5), centrifuged at 16,000 g for 25 min, washed in ice-cold buffer, and re-centrifuged. The washing procedure was repeated four times and the membrane pellet stored at -80° C until use. Tissue pellets were re-suspended in ice-cold binding buffer (10 mmol NaH_2PO_4, 10 mmol Na_2HPO_4, 1 mmol $MgCl_2$, pH = 7.4) and protein concentrations measured (BCA protein assay kit, Pierce, Rockford IL).

Tissue samples (50 μL) were incubated for 1 hour in triplicate (hippocampus) or duplicate (cortex) in a total volume of 200 μL, containing binding buffer (50 μL), radioligand (50 μL), and 2.5 mmol atropine to measure nonspecific binding or water (50 μL). Single point saturation binding was performed for hippocampal preparations due to the limited amount of tissue (98 nM [^{3}H] pirenzepine and 85 nM [^{3}H] AF-DX-384). For the cortical binding, eight different increasing concentrations of [^{3}H] pirenzepine (330 pM - 46 nM) or [^{3}H] AF-DX-384 (252 pM - 46 nM) were used. Following incubation, 5 mL of ice-cold binding buffer was added to stop the reaction and tissues were bound to filter paper (Beckman, Fullerton, CA) using a cell harvester (Brandel, Gaithersburg, MD). Filters were placed in vials and 5 mL of scintillation fluid (Optiphase 2, Perkin Elmer, Waltham, MA) was added before counting radioactivity using a beta counter (LS 6000SC, Beta Counter, Beckman). The maximal number of binding sites (B_{max}) and the equilibrium dissociation constant (K_d, for cortical binding only) were determined according to the Hill equation (Whiteaker, Jimenez, McIntosh, Collins, & Marks, 2000) using nonlinear regression analysis and Graphpad Prism 4.0 software (Graphpad, San Diego, CA).

A two-way ANOVA was used to assess the effects of treatment and sex on the B_{max} and K_d of the mAChRs in the hippocampus and cortex. In the hippocampus, MA-exposed mice had a higher number (B_{max}) of M_1 mAChRs compared to SA-exposed mice (F (1, 15) = 4.63, $p = 0.04$; Table 4). Female mice had a higher number of M_1 mAChRs compared to male mice (F (1, 16) = 7.45, $p = 0.02$; Table 4). There was no effect of treatment or sex on the number of M_2 mAChRs in the hippocampus (Table 4). In the cortex, there was no effect of treatment or sex on the number or dissociation constant (K_d) of either the M_1 or M_2 mAChRs (data not shown).

Table 4. Summary of the number (B_{max}) of muscarinic receptors in the hippocampus of adolescent mice

Treatment	Sex	M_1 mAChRs	M_2 mAChRs
SA	Males	1126.7 ± 51.2	2463.6 ± 92.2
MA	Males	1308.6 ± 101.9*	2503.2 ± 99.1
SA	Females	1359.8 ± 75.8[a]	2357.9 ± 127.0
MA	Females	1559.1 ± 95.4*[a]	1234.1 ± 47.9

* MA-exposed mice higher than SA-exposed mice, $p < 0.05$ main effect of treatment.
[a] Female mice higher than male mice, $p < 0.05$ main effect of sex.

These results show a sex-dependent effect of MA on the cholinergic system; female adolescent mice had increased cholinergic cell density in the MS/VDB/HDB and ChAT-positive fibers in the hippocampus following MA exposure, whereas these effects were not seen in males. However, both male and female mice showed an increase in M_1 mAChR binding in the hippocampus. The sex dependency is striking based on the increased susceptibility of female mice to the developmental effects of MA on cognition described earlier. The mechanism underlying these sex-dependent effects is unknown. Female mice show higher concentrations of MA in the cortex 120 minutes following single injection of MA (5 mg/kg) on PD 11 compared to male mice (Acevedo et al., 2008). Female mice also show a trend toward higher MA concentrations in the cortex and hippocampus on PD 15 and 20 compared to male mice one hour post MA injections from PD 11-20. Thus, female mice might metabolize MA in the brain at a slower rate than male mice. The slower metabolism of MA in female mice may increase MA-induced neurotoxicity on the ACh system. Alternatively or in addition, the sex-dependent effects of MA on the cholinergic system could be due in part to sex differences in the timeline of cholinergic development. ChAT activity levels in the MS mature earlier in female rats, while male rats show increases in ChAT activity after PD 18 (Loy & Sheldon, 1987). Thus MA exposure from PD 11-20 may target a sensitive period of ChAT development in female but not male mice.

Increased mAChRs in both male and female adolescent mice suggest that MA has effects in male mice, but they are more limited compared to those in female mice. MA exposure decreased the density of cholinergic cells in the male mice as opposed to the increase seen in female mice, although these changes did not reach statistical significance. However, this finding parallels a decrease seen in AChE-positive fibers in the hippocampus of adult male gerbils following postnatal MA exposure (Busche et al., 2006). MA-induced decreases in cholinergic cells may result in a compensatory up-regulation of mAChRs in the hippocampus in male mice. Female mice also showed a MA-induced increase in hippocampal mAChRs, suggesting that different mechanisms may underlie this effect in males and females.

The precise mechanism by which MA affects the cholinergic system is not yet understood. The time period of MA exposure (PD 11-20) overlaps with important aspects of cholinergic BF development in rodents, including developmental increases in ChAT and AChE activity and mAChR levels in the BF, hippocampus, and cortex (Aubert et al., 1996; Berse et al., 2005; Kiss & Patel, 1992; Thal et al., 1992; Zahalka et al., 1993). MA-induced increases in cholinergic cell density in the MS/VDB/HDB of female mice could arise by MA-induced enhancement of cholinergic differentiation of proliferating precursor cells, by increased cholinergic cell survival, or by enhancement of the cholinergic phenotype within differentiated cholinergic cells. It is unlikely that MA exposure from PD 11-20 affects differentiation of proliferating precursor cells, as the BF cholinergic neurons divide and migrate before birth (Brady et al., 1989; Schambra et al., 1989). MA exposure also does not promote overall increases in new neurons, as there was no increase in total neuronal density, suggesting no effects on cell survival. MA exposure may have increased cholinergic phenotype expression within cholinergic neurons from basal levels, or induced a switch from another phenotype to the cholinergic phenotype. The BF contains GABAergic and glutamatergic neurons in addition to the cholinergic neurons (Gritti et al., 2003). There was no change in GABAergic cells, and if anything, MA exposure in the female mice increased the density of GABAergic cells, suggesting that MA did not induce a phenotype change from GABAergic to cholinergic. Although there was no significant decrease in percent of non-cholinergic or GABAergic (presumably glutamatergic) "other" neurons, MA-exposed female mice did show a lower percent of "other" neurons and an increase in cholinergic neurons compared to SA-exposed female mice (data not shown). A very small reduction in the percent of "other" neurons could contribute to a significant change in the percent of cholinergic cells, as the percentage of the cholinergic cells was quite low compared to the other phenotypes. Thus while a significant reduction in "other" neurons was not observed, there could have been a small

MA-induced change in phenotype toward a detectable increase in the cholinergic phenotype. Further research is needed to quantify the density of glutamatergic neurons in addition to cholinergic and GABAergic neurons to determine MA-induced changes in this neuronal population.

There was no effect of MA exposure on the density of NB cholinergic neurons. In parallel with this finding, there was also no increase in the area occupied by cholinergic fibers in any region of the cortex examined. As the NB is the primary source of cholinergic innervation in the cortex (Mesulam et al., 1983), these findings are consistent with the region-specific effects of MA exposure in the BF. Similarly there were no changes in cortical mAChRs, again suggesting specific effects of MA on the MS/VDB/HDB and the corresponding projections to the hippocampus. These findings imply that the effects of MA in the MS/VDB/HDB are linked to those in the hippocampus, and that these MA-induced alterations might contribute to MA-induced cognitive impairments on hippocampus-dependent tasks (Acevedo et al., 2007; Siegel et al., 2010; Siegel, Park et al., 2011).

Conclusion

The data described in this chapter support the involvement of the histaminergic and cholinergic systems in mediating the effects of neonatal MA exposure on hippocampal function and hippocampus-dependent cognition during adolescence and adulthood. For several, but not all, outcome measures, females are more susceptible than males to MA exposure during hippocampal development. Increased efforts are warranted to determine the mechanisms underlying these detrimental effects of MA and the mechanisms that might be targeted therapeutically to reduce or even prevent these MA-induced effects.

Acknowledgment

This work was supported by the National Institute of Drug Abuse Training Grant T32DA07262, National Research Service Award F31DA026243, the Methamphetamine Abuse Research Center Grant 1P50DA018165, an Achievement Rewards for College Scientists (ARCS) Scholarship, and the development account of Dr. Raber. The authors would like to thank Emily

Eastwood for breeding, injecting, and testing adolescent mice in the water maze following neonatal MA or THIO exposure.

References

Abreu-Villaca, Y., Filgueiras, C. C., & Manhaes, A. C. (2010). Developmental aspects of the cholinergic system. *Behav Brain Res.*

Acevedo, S. F., de Esch, I. J., & Raber, J. (2007). Sex- and histamine-dependent long-term cognitive effects of methamphetamine exposure. *Neuropsychopharmacology, 32*(3), 665-672.

Acevedo, S. F., Pfankuch, T., van Meer, P., & Raber, J. (2008). Role of histamine in short- and long-term effects of methamphetamine on the developing mouse brain. *J Neurochem, 107*(4), 976-986.

Arnold, H. M., Burk, J. A., Hodgson, E. M., Sarter, M., & Bruno, J. P. (2002). Differential cortical acetylcholine release in rats performing a sustained attention task versus behavioral control tasks that do not explicitly tax attention. *Neuroscience, 114*(2), 451-460.

Arrang, J. M., Garbarg, M., & Schwartz, J. C. (1983). Auto-inhibition of brain histamine release mediated by a novel class (H3) of histamine receptor. *Nature, 302*(5911), 832-837.

Arters, J., Hohmann, C. F., Mills, J., Olaghere, O., & Berger-Sweeney, J. (1998). Sexually dimorphic responses to neonatal basal forebrain lesions in mice: I. Behavior and neurochemistry. *Journal of Neurobiology, 37*(4), 582-594.

Aubert, I., Cecyre, D., Gauthier, S., & Quirion, R. (1992). Characterization and autoradiographic distribution of [3H]AF-DX 384 binding to putative muscarinic M2 receptors in the rat brain. *Eur J Pharmacol, 217*(2-3), 173-184.

Aubert, I., Cecyre, D., Gauthier, S., & Quirion, R. (1996). Comparative ontogenic profile of cholinergic markers, including nicotinic and muscarinic receptors, in the rat brain. *J Comp Neurol, 369*(1), 31-55.

Auvinen, S., & Panula, P. (1988). Development of histamine-immunoreactive neurons in the rat brain. *J Comp Neurol, 276*(2), 289-303.

Barr, A. M., Panenka, W. J., MacEwan, G. W., Thornton, A. E., Lang, D. J., Honer, W. G., et al. (2006). The need for speed: an update on methamphetamine addiction. *J Psychiatry Neurosci, 31*(5), 301-313.

Berger-Sweeney, J. (2003). The cholinergic basal forebrain system during development and its influence on cognitive processes: important questions and potential answers. *Neurosci Biobehav Rev, 27*(4), 401-411.

Berse, B., Szczecinska, W., Lopez-Coviella, I., Madziar, B., Zemelko, V., Kaminski, R., et al. (2005). Expression of high affinity choline transporter during mouse development in vivo and its upregulation by NGF and BMP-4 in vitro. *Brain Res Dev Brain Res, 157*(2), 132-140.

Bockaert, J., & Pin, J. P. (1999). Molecular tinkering of G protein-coupled receptors: an evolutionary success. *EMBO J, 18*(7), 1723-1729.

Bongers, G., Leurs, R., Robertson, J., & Raber, J. (2004). Role of H3-receptor-mediated signaling in anxiety and cognition in wild-type and Apoe-/- mice. *Neuropsychopharmacology, 29*(3), 441-449.

Brady, D. R., Phelps, P. E., & Vaughn, J. E. (1989). Neurogenesis of basal forebrain cholinergic neurons in rat. *Brain Res Dev Brain Res, 47*(1), 81-92.

Bredy, T. W., Lee, A. W., Meaney, M. J., & Brown, R. E. (2004). Effect of neonatal handling and paternal care on offspring cognitive development in the monogamous California mouse (Peromyscus californicus). *Horm Behav, 46*(1), 30-38.

Broening, H. W., Pu, C., & Vorhees, C. V. (1997). Methamphetamine selectively damages dopaminergic innervation to the nucleus accumbens core while sparing the shell. *Synapse, 27*(2), 153-160.

Brown, R. E., Stevens, D. R., & Haas, H. L. (2001). The physiology of brain histamine. *Prog Neurobiol, 63*(6), 637-672.

Busche, A., Bagorda, A., Lehmann, K., Neddens, J., & Teuchert-Noodt, G. (2006). The maturation of the acetylcholine system in the dentate gyrus of gerbils (Meriones unguiculatus) is affected by epigenetic factors. *J Neural Transm, 113*(2), 113-124.

Chang, L., Cloak, C., Jiang, C. S., Farnham, S., Tokeshi, B., Buchthal, S., et al. (2009). Altered neurometabolites and motor integration in children exposed to methamphetamine in utero. *Neuroimage, 48*(2), 391-397.

Chang, L., Smith, L. M., LoPresti, C., Yonekura, M. L., Kuo, J., Walot, I., et al. (2004). Smaller subcortical volumes and cognitive deficits in children with prenatal methamphetamine exposure. *Psychiatry Res, 132*(2), 95-106.

Clancy, B., Finlay, B. L., Darlington, R. B., & Anand, K. J. (2007). Extrapolating brain development from experimental species to humans. *Neurotoxicology, 28*(5), 931-937.

Clancy, B., Kersh, B., Hyde, J., Darlington, R. B., Anand, K. J., & Finlay, B. L. (2007). Web-Based Method For Translating Neurodevelopment From Laboratory Species To Humans. *Neuroinformatics, 5*(1), 79-94.

Clark, E. A., & Hill, S. J. (1996). Sensitivity of histamine H3 receptor agonist-stimulated [35S]GTP gamma[S] binding to pertussis toxin. *Eur J Pharmacol, 296*(2), 223-225.

Coge, F., Guenin, S. P., Rique, H., Boutin, J. A., & Galizzi, J. P. (2001). Structure and expression of the human histamine H4-receptor gene. *Biochem Biophys Res Commun, 284*(2), 301-309.

Cruickshank, C. C., & Dyer, K. R. (2009). A review of the clinical pharmacology of methamphetamine. *Addiction, 104*(7), 1085-1099.

Cummings, J. L. (2000). Cholinesterase inhibitors: A new class of psychotropic compounds. *Am J Psychiatry, 157*(1), 4-15.

Dai, H., Okuda, H., Iwabuchi, K., Sakurai, E., Chen, Z., Kato, M., et al. (2004). Social isolation stress significantly enhanced the disruption of prepulse inhibition in mice repeatedly treated with methamphetamine. *Ann N Y Acad Sci, 1025*, 257-266.

Dai, H., Okuda, T., Sakurai, E., Kuramasu, A., Kato, M., Jia, F., et al. (2005). Blockage of histamine H1 receptor attenuates social isolation-induced disruption of prepulse inhibition: a study in H1 receptor gene knockout mice. *Psychopharmacology (Berl), 183*(3), 285-293.

Dalley, J. W., McGaughy, J., O'Connell, M. T., Cardinal, R. N., Levita, L., & Robbins, T. W. (2001). Distinct changes in cortical acetylcholine and noradrenaline efflux during contingent and noncontingent performance of a visual attentional task. *J Neurosci, 21*(13), 4908-4914.

DASIS. (2008). The Drug and Alcohol Services Information System Report: Primary Methamphetamine/Amphetamine Admissions to Substance Abuse Treatment 1-4.

DAWN. (2010). The Drug Abuse Warning Network Report: Emergency Department Visits Involving Methamphetamine from http://www.oas.samhsa.gov/2k10/DAWN017/Meth.htm

DEA. (2006). General information regarding "The Combat Methamphetamine Epidemic Act of 2005". 1-8.

Deacon, R. M., Bannerman, D. M., Kirby, B. P., Croucher, A., & Rawlins, J. N. (2002). Effects of cytotoxic hippocampal lesions in mice on a cognitive test battery. *Behav Brain Res, 133*(1), 57-68.

Decker, M. W., Majchrzak, M. J., & Anderson, D. J. (1992). Effects of nicotine on spatial memory deficits in rats with septal lesions. *Brain Res, 572*(1-2), 281-285.

Dobbs, L. K., & Mark, G. P. (2008). Comparison of systemic and local methamphetamine treatment on acetylcholine and dopamine levels in the ventral tegmental area in the mouse. *Neuroscience, 156*(3), 700-711.

Feiro, O., & Gould, T. J. (2005). The interactive effects of nicotinic and muscarinic cholinergic receptor inhibition on fear conditioning in young and aged C57BL/6 mice. *Pharmacol Biochem Behav, 80*(2), 251-262.

Feldman, R. S., Meyer, J. S., & Quenzer, L. F. (1997). *Principles of Neuropsychopharmacology*. Sunderland: Sinauer Associates, Inc.

Fontana, D. J., Inouye, G. T., & Johnson, R. M. (1994). Linopirdine (DuP 996) improves performance in several tests of learning and memory by modulation of cholinergic neurotransmission. *Pharmacol Biochem Behav, 49*(4), 1075-1082.

Franklin, K., & Paxinos, G. (1997). *The mouse brain in stereotaxic coordinates*. San Diego: Academic Press.

Freund, T. F. (1989). GABAergic septohippocampal neurons contain parvalbumin. *Brain Res, 478*(2), 375-381.

Freund, T. F., & Antal, M. (1988). GABA-containing neurons in the septum control inhibitory interneurons in the hippocampus. *Nature, 336*(6195), 170-173.

Freund, T. F., & Meskenaite, V. (1992). gamma-Aminobutyric acid-containing basal forebrain neurons innervate inhibitory interneurons in the neocortex. *Proc Natl Acad Sci U S A, 89*(2), 738-742.

Frick, K. M., Kim, J. J., & Baxter, M. G. (2004). Effects of complete immunotoxin lesions of the cholinergic basal forebrain on fear conditioning and spatial learning. *Hippocampus, 14*(2), 244-254.

Froeliger, B., Gilbert, D. G., & McClernon, F. J. (2009). Effects of nicotine on novelty detection and memory recognition performance: double-blind, placebo-controlled studies of smokers and nonsmokers. *Psychopharmacology (Berl), 205*(4), 625-633.

Garcia-Rates, S., Camarasa, J., Escubedo, E., & Pubill, D. (2007). Methamphetamine and 3,4-methylenedioxymethamphetamine interact with central nicotinic receptors and induce their up-regulation. *Toxicol Appl Pharmacol, 223*(3), 195-205.

Garcia, M., Floran, B., Arias-Montano, J. A., Young, J. M., & Aceves, J. (1997). Histamine H3 receptor activation selectively inhibits dopamine D1 receptor-dependent [3H]GABA release from depolarization-stimulated slices of rat substantia nigra pars reticulata. *Neuroscience, 80*(1), 241-249.

Gaykema, R. P., Luiten, P. G., Nyakas, C., & Traber, J. (1990). Cortical projection patterns of the medial septum-diagonal band complex. *J Comp Neurol, 293*(1), 103-124.

Gerlai, R. T., McNamara, A., Williams, S., & Phillips, H. S. (2002). Hippocampal dysfunction and behavioral deficit in the water maze in mice: an unresolved issue? *Brain Res Bull, 57*(1), 3-9.

Gettig, J. P., Grady, S. E., & Nowosadzka, I. (2006). Methamphetamine: putting the brakes on speed. *J Sch Nurs, 22*(2), 66-73.

Ghi, P., Orsetti, M., Gamalero, S. R., & Ferretti, C. (1999). Sex differences in memory performance in the object recognition test. Possible role of histamine receptors. *Pharmacol Biochem Behav, 64*(4), 761-766.

Gilman, A. G., Rall, T. W., Nies, A. S., & Taylor, P. (Eds.). (1993). *Goodman and Gilman's the pharmacological basis of therapeutics* (Eighth ed.). New York: McGraw-Hill, INC.

Giovannini, M. G., Bartolini, L., Bacciottini, L., Greco, L., & Blandina, P. (1999). Effects of histamine H3 receptor agonists and antagonists on cognitive performance and scopolamine-induced amnesia. *Behav Brain Res, 104*(1-2), 147-155.

Gonzales, R., Mooney, L., & Rawson, R. A. (2010). The methamphetamine problem in the United States. *Annu Rev Public Health, 31*, 385-398.

Good, M. M., Solt, I., Acuna, J. G., Rotmensch, S., & Kim, M. J. (2010). Methamphetamine use during pregnancy: maternal and neonatal implications. *Obstet Gynecol, 116*(2 Pt 1), 330-334.

Gritti, I., Mainville, L., & Jones, B. E. (1993). Codistribution of GABA- with acetylcholine-synthesizing neurons in the basal forebrain of the rat. *J Comp Neurol, 329*(4), 438-457.

Gritti, I., Mainville, L., & Jones, B. E. (1994). Projections of GABAergic and cholinergic basal forebrain and GABAergic preoptic-anterior hypothalamic neurons to the posterior lateral hypothalamus of the rat. *J Comp Neurol, 339*(2), 251-268.

Gritti, I., Manns, I. D., Mainville, L., & Jones, B. E. (2003). Parvalbumin, calbindin, or calretinin in cortically projecting and GABAergic, cholinergic, or glutamatergic basal forebrain neurons of the rat. *J Comp Neurol, 458*(1), 11-31.

Guilarte, T. R., Nihei, M. K., McGlothan, J. L., & Howard, A. S. (2003). Methamphetamine-induced deficits of brain monoaminergic neuronal markers: distal axotomy or neuronal plasticity. *Neuroscience, 122*(2), 499-513.

Halbach, O., & Dermietzel, H. (2002). *Neurotransmitters and Neuromodulators: Handbook of Receptors and Biological Effects* (Vol. 1). Weinheim: Wiley-VCH.

Hellstrom-Lindahl, E., Gorbounova, O., Seiger, A., Mousavi, M., & Nordberg, A. (1998). Regional distribution of nicotinic receptors during prenatal development of human brain and spinal cord. *Brain Res Dev Brain Res, 108*(1-2), 147-160.

Henny, P., & Jones, B. E. (2006). Innervation of orexin/hypocretin neurons by GABAergic, glutamatergic or cholinergic basal forebrain terminals evidenced by immunostaining for presynaptic vesicular transporter and postsynaptic scaffolding proteins. *J Comp Neurol, 499*(4), 645-661.

Hill, S. J., Ganellin, C. R., Timmerman, H., Schwartz, J. C., Shankley, N. P., Young, J. M., et al. (1997). International Union of Pharmacology. XIII. Classification of histamine receptors. *Pharmacol Rev, 49*(3), 253-278.

Himmelheber, A. M., Sarter, M., & Bruno, J. P. (2000). Increases in cortical acetylcholine release during sustained attention performance in rats. *Brain Res Cogn Brain Res, 9*(3), 313-325.

Hoffman, W. F., Moore, M., Templin, R., McFarland, B., Hitzemann, R. J., & Mitchell, S. H. (2006). Neuropsychological function and delay discounting in methamphetamine-dependent individuals. *Psychopharmacology (Berl), 188*(2), 162-170.

Houser, C. R., Crawford, G. D., Barber, R. P., Salvaterra, P. M., & Vaughn, J. E. (1983). Organization and morphological characteristics of cholinergic neurons: an immunocytochemical study with a monoclonal antibody to choline acetyltransferase. *Brain Res, 266*(1), 97-119.

Hussain, R. J., Taraschenko, O. D., & Glick, S. D. (2008). Effects of nicotine, methamphetamine and cocaine on extracellular levels of acetylcholine in the interpeduncular nucleus of rats. *Neurosci Lett, 440*(3), 270-274.

Huston, J. P., Wagner, U., & Hasenohrl, R. U. (1997). The tuberomammillary nucleus projections in the control of learning, memory and reinforcement processes: evidence for an inhibitory role. *Behav Brain Res, 83*(1-2), 97-105.

Ito, C., Onodera, K., Watanabe, T., & Sato, M. (1997). Effects of histamine agents on methamphetamine-induced stereotyped behavior and behavioral sensitization in rats. *Psychopharmacology (Berl), 130*(4), 362-367.

Izumi, H., Makino, Y., Shirakawa, K., & Garfield, R. E. (1995). Role of nitric oxide on vasorelaxation in human umbilical artery. *Am J Obstet Gynecol, 172*(5), 1477-1484.

Jansen, F. P., Mochizuki, T., Yamamoto, Y., Timmerman, H., & Yamatodani, A. (1998). In vivo modulation of rat hypothalamic histamine release by the histamine H3 receptor ligands, immepip and clobenpropit. Effects of intrahypothalamic and peripheral application. *Eur J Pharmacol, 362*(2-3), 149-155.

Johanson, C. E., Frey, K. A., Lundahl, L. H., Keenan, P., Lockhart, N., Roll, J., et al. (2006). Cognitive function and nigrostriatal markers in abstinent methamphetamine abusers. *Psychopharmacology (Berl), 185*(3), 327-338.

Jones, C. K., & Shannon, H. E. (2000). Muscarinic cholinergic modulation of prepulse inhibition of the acoustic startle reflex. *J Pharmacol Exp Ther, 294*(3), 1017-1023.

Karlstedt, K., Ahman, M. J., Anichtchik, O. V., Soinila, S., & Panula, P. (2003). Expression of the H3 receptor in the developing CNS and brown fat suggests novel roles for histamine. *Mol Cell Neurosci, 24*(3), 614-622.

Katzung, B. G. (2007). *Basic and Clinical Pharmacology* (10th ed.). New York: McGraw-Hill Companies, Inc.

Kinnunen, A., Lintunen, M., Karlstedt, K., Fukui, H., & Panula, P. (1998). In situ detection of H1-receptor mRNA and absence of apoptosis in the transient histamine system of the embryonic rat brain. *J Comp Neurol, 394*(1), 127-137.

Kish, S. J., Kalasinsky, K. S., Furukawa, Y., Guttman, M., Ang, L., Li, L., et al. (1999). Brain choline acetyltransferase activity in chronic, human users of cocaine, methamphetamine, and heroin. *Mol Psychiatry, 4*(1), 26-32.

Kiss, J., & Patel, A. J. (1992). Development of the cholinergic fibres innervating the cerebral cortex of the rat. *Int J Dev Neurosci, 10*(2), 153-170.

Kiss, J., Patel, A. J., Baimbridge, K. G., & Freund, T. F. (1990). Topographical localization of neurons containing parvalbumin and choline acetyltransferase in the medial septum-diagonal band region of the rat. *Neuroscience, 36*(1), 61-72.

Lehmann, K., Hundsdorfer, B., Hartmann, T., & Teuchert-Noodt, G. (2004). The acetylcholine fiber density of the neocortex is altered by isolated rearing and early methamphetamine intoxication in rodents. *Exp Neurol, 189*(1), 131-140.

Lester, B. M., & Lagasse, L. L. (2010). Children of addicted women. *J Addict Dis, 29*(2), 259-276.

Li, H., Burkhardt, C., Heinrich, U. R., Brausch, I., Xia, N., & Forstermann, U. (2003). Histamine upregulates gene expression of endothelial nitric oxide synthase in human vascular endothelial cells. *Circulation, 107*(18), 2348-2354.

Lin, L., LeBlanc, C. J., Deacon, T. W., & Isacson, O. (1998). Chronic cognitive deficits and amyloid precursor protein elevation after selective immunotoxin lesions of the basal forebrain cholinergic system. *Neuroreport, 9*(3), 547-552.

Linke, R., Schwegler, H., & Boldyreva, M. (1994). Cholinergic and GABAergic septo-hippocampal projection neurons in mice: a retrograde tracing study combined with double immunocytochemistry for choline acetyltransferase and parvalbumin. *Brain Res, 653*(1-2), 73-80.

Little, B. B., Snell, L. M., & Gilstrap, L. C., 3rd. (1988). Methamphetamine abuse during pregnancy: outcome and fetal effects. *Obstet Gynecol, 72*(4), 541-544.

Lovenberg, T. W., Roland, B. L., Wilson, S. J., Jiang, X., Pyati, J., Huvar, A., et al. (1999). Cloning and functional expression of the human histamine H3 receptor. *Mol Pharmacol, 55*(6), 1101-1107.

Loy, R., & Sheldon, R. A. (1987). Sexually dimorphic development of cholinergic enzymes in the rat septohippocampal system. *Brain Res, 431*(1), 156-160.

Lu, L. H., Johnson, A., O'Hare, E. D., Bookheimer, S. Y., Smith, L. M., O'Connor, M. J., et al. (2009). Effects of prenatal methamphetamine exposure on verbal memory revealed with functional magnetic resonance imaging. *J Dev Behav Pediatr, 30*(3), 185-192.

Manns, I. D., Mainville, L., & Jones, B. E. (2001). Evidence for glutamate, in addition to acetylcholine and GABA, neurotransmitter synthesis in basal forebrain neurons projecting to the entorhinal cortex. *Neuroscience, 107*(2), 249-263.

McCabe, R. T., Gibb, J. W., Wamsley, J. K., & Hanson, G. R. (1987). Autoradiographic analysis of muscarinic cholinergic and serotonergic receptor alterations following methamphetamine treatment. *Brain Res Bull, 19*(5), 551-557.

McCabe, R. T., Hanson, G. R., Dawson, T. M., Wamsley, J. K., & Gibb, J. W. (1987). Methamphetamine-induced reduction in D1 and D2 dopamine receptors as evidenced by autoradiography: comparison with tyrosine hydroxylase activity. *Neuroscience, 23*(1), 253-261.

Mesulam, M. M. (2004). The cholinergic innervation of the human cerebral cortex. *Prog Brain Res, 145*, 67-78.

Mesulam, M. M., Mufson, E. J., Wainer, B. H., & Levey, A. I. (1983). Central cholinergic pathways in the rat: an overview based on an alternative nomenclature (Ch1-Ch6). *Neuroscience, 10*(4), 1185-1201.

Mirza, N. R., & Stolerman, I. P. (2000). The role of nicotinic and muscarinic acetylcholine receptors in attention. *Psychopharmacology (Berl), 148*(3), 243-250.

Miyazaki, S., Onodera, K., Imaizumi, M., & Timmerman, H. (1997). Effects of clobenpropit (VUF-9153), a histamine H3-receptor antagonist, on learning and memory, and on cholinergic and monoaminergic systems in mice. *Life Sci, 61*(4), 355-361.

Mori, T., Narita, M., Onodera, K., & Suzuki, T. (2002). Modulation of the discriminative stimulus effects of cocaine and methamphetamine by the histaminergic system. *Nihon Shinkei Seishin Yakurigaku Zasshi, 22*(3), 73-78.

Morris, R. G., Garrud, P., Rawlins, J. N., & O'Keefe, J. (1982). Place navigation impaired in rats with hippocampal lesions. *Nature, 297*(5868), 681-683.

Muir, J. L., Everitt, B. J., & Robbins, T. W. (1994). AMPA-induced excitotoxic lesions of the basal forebrain: a significant role for the cortical cholinergic system in attentional function. *J Neurosci, 14*(4), 2313-2326.

Mullen, R. J., Buck, C. R., & Smith, A. M. (1992). NeuN, a neuronal specific nuclear protein in vertebrates. *Development, 116*(1), 201-211.

Mumby, D. G., Gaskin, S., Glenn, M. J., Schramek, T. E., & Lehmann, H. (2002). Hippocampal damage and exploratory preferences in rats: memory for objects, places, and contexts. *Learn Mem, 9*(2), 49-57.

Munzar, P., Nosal, R., & Goldberg, S. R. (1998). Potentiation of the discriminative-stimulus effects of methamphetamine by the histamine H3 receptor antagonist thioperamide in rats. *Eur J Pharmacol, 363*(2-3), 93-101.

Munzar, P., Tanda, G., Justinova, Z., & Goldberg, S. R. (2004). Histamine h3 receptor antagonists potentiate methamphetamine self-administration and methamphetamine-induced accumbal dopamine release. *Neuropsychopharmacology, 29*(4), 705-717.

Murai, T., Okuda, S., Tanaka, T., & Ohta, H. (2007). Characteristics of object location memory in mice: Behavioral and pharmacological studies. *Physiol Behav, 90*(1), 116-124.

Nail-Boucherie, K., Dourmap, N., Jaffard, R., & Costentin, J. (2000). Contextual fear conditioning is associated with an increase of acetylcholine release in the hippocampus of rat. *Brain Res Cogn Brain Res, 9*(2), 193-197.

Nakamura, T., Itadani, H., Hidaka, Y., Ohta, M., & Tanaka, K. (2000). Molecular cloning and characterization of a new human histamine receptor, HH4R. *Biochem Biophys Res Commun, 279*(2), 615-620.

NIDA. (2006). Research Report Series : Methamphetamine Abuse and Addiction. 1-8.

NIDA. (2010). InfoFacts: Methamphetamine. 1-4.

NSDUH. (2007). The National Survey on Drug Use and Health Report: Methamphetamine Use. 1-4.

NSDUH. (2009). Results from the 2009 National Survey on Drug Use and Health: Volume I. Summary of National Findings. 1-104.

Oda, Y. (1999). Choline acetyltransferase: the structure, distribution and pathologic changes in the central nervous system. *Pathol Int, 49*(11), 921-937.

Otto, T., & Poon, P. (2006). Dorsal hippocampal contributions to unimodal contextual conditioning. *J Neurosci, 26*(24), 6603-6609.

Pappas, B. A., Payne, K. B., Fortin, T., & Sherren, N. (2005). Neonatal lesion of forebrain cholinergic neurons: further characterization of behavioral effects and permanency. *Neuroscience, 133*(2), 485-492.

Passetti, F., Dalley, J. W., O'Connell, M. T., Everitt, B. J., & Robbins, T. W. (2000). Increased acetylcholine release in the rat medial prefrontal cortex during performance of a visual attentional task. *Eur J Neurosci, 12*(8), 3051-3058.

Paterson, D., & Nordberg, A. (2000). Neuronal nicotinic receptors in the human brain. *Prog Neurobiol, 61*(1), 75-111.

Paz, M. S., Smith, L. M., LaGasse, L. L., Derauf, C., Grant, P., Shah, R., et al. (2009). Maternal depression and neurobehavior in newborns prenatally exposed to methamphetamine. *Neurotoxicol Teratol, 31*(3), 177-182.

Phillips, J. M., McAlonan, K., Robb, W. G., & Brown, V. J. (2000). Cholinergic neurotransmission influences covert orientation of visuospatial attention in the rat. *Psychopharmacology (Berl), 150*(1), 112-116.

Phillips, R. G., & LeDoux, J. E. (1992). Differential contribution of amygdala and hippocampus to cued and contextual fear conditioning. *Behav Neurosci, 106*(2), 274-285.

Piper, B. J., Acevedo, S. F., Kolchugina, G. K., Butler, R. W., Corbett, S. M., Honeycutt, E. B., et al. (2011). Abnormalities in parentally rated executive function in methamphetamine/polysubstance exposed children. *Pharmacol Biochem Behav, 98*, 432-439.

Prast, H., Argyriou, A., & Philippu, A. (1996). Histaminergic neurons facilitate social memory in rats. *Brain Res, 734*(1-2), 316-318.

Ravikumar, B. V., & Sastry, P. S. (1985). Muscarinic cholinergic receptors in human foetal brain: characterization and ontogeny of [3H]quinuclidinyl benzilate binding sites in frontal cortex. *J Neurochem, 44*(1), 240-246.

Ricceri, L., Hohmann, C., & Berger-Sweeney, J. (2002). Early neonatal 192 IgG saporin induces learning impairments and disrupts cortical morphogenesis in rats. *Brain Res, 954*(2), 160-172.

Ricceri, L., Minghetti, L., Moles, A., Popoli, P., Confaloni, A., De Simone, R., et al. (2004). Cognitive and neurological deficits induced by early and prolonged basal forebrain cholinergic hypofunction in rats. *Exp Neurol, 189*(1), 162-172.

Rice, C. J., Sandman, C. A., Lenjavi, M. R., & Baram, T. Z. (2008). A novel mouse model for acute and long-lasting consequences of early life stress. *Endocrinology, 149*(10), 4892-4900.

Risbrough, V., Bontempi, B., & Menzaghi, F. (2002). Selective immune-lesioning of the basal forebrain cholinergic neurons in rats: effect on attention using the 5-choice serial reaction time task. *Psychopharmacology (Berl), 164*(1), 71-81.

Robbins, T. W. (2002). The 5-choice serial reaction time task: behavioural pharmacology and functional neurochemistry. *Psychopharmacology (Berl), 163*(3-4), 362-380.

Rogers, J. L., & Kesner, R. P. (2004). Cholinergic modulation of the hippocampus during encoding and retrieval of tone/shock-induced fear conditioning. *Learn Mem, 11*(1), 102-107.

Rubio, S., Begega, A., Santin, L. J., & Arias, J. L. (2002). Improvement of spatial memory by (R)-alpha-methylhistamine, a histamine H(3)-receptor agonist, on the Morris water-maze in rat. *Behav Brain Res, 129*(1-2), 77-82.

Ruotsalainen, S., Miettinen, R., MacDonald, E., Koivisto, E., & Sirvio, J. (2000). Blockade of muscarinic, rather than nicotinic, receptors impairs attention, but does not interact with serotonin depletion. *Psychopharmacology (Berl), 148*(2), 111-123.

Ryu, J. H., Yanai, K., Sakurai, E., Kim, C. Y., & Watanabe, T. (1995). Ontogenetic development of histamine receptor subtypes in rat brain demonstrated by quantitative autoradiography. *Brain Res Dev Brain Res, 87*(2), 101-110.

Sambeth, A., Riedel, W. J., Smits, L. T., & Blokland, A. (2007). Cholinergic drugs affect novel object recognition in rats: relation with hippocampal EEG? *Eur J Pharmacol, 572*(2-3), 151-159.

Save, E., Poucet, B., Foreman, N., & Buhot, M. C. (1992). Object exploration and reactions to spatial and nonspatial changes in hooded rats following damage to parietal cortex or hippocampal formation. *Behav Neurosci, 106*(3), 447-456.

Schambra, U. B., Sulik, K. K., Petrusz, P., & Lauder, J. M. (1989). Ontogeny of cholinergic neurons in the mouse forebrain. *J Comp Neurol, 288*(1), 101-122.

Schlicker, E., Betz, R., & Gothert, M. (1988). Histamine H3 receptor-mediated inhibition of serotonin release in the rat brain cortex. *Naunyn Schmiedebergs Arch Pharmacol, 337*(5), 588-590.

Schlicker, E., Fink, K., Detzner, M., & Gothert, M. (1993). Histamine inhibits dopamine release in the mouse striatum via presynaptic H3 receptors. *J Neural Transm Gen Sect, 93*(1), 1-10.

Schlicker, E., Schunack, W., & Gothert, M. (1990). Histamine H3 receptor-mediated inhibition of noradrenaline release in pig retina discs. *Naunyn Schmiedebergs Arch Pharmacol, 342*(5), 497-501.

Schwab, C., Bruckner, G., Rothe, T., Castellano, C., & Oliverio, A. (1992). Autoradiography of muscarinic cholinergic receptors in cortical and subcortical brain regions of C57BL/6 and DBA/2 mice. *Neurochem Res, 17*(11), 1057-1062.

Scott, J. C., Woods, S. P., Matt, G. E., Meyer, R. A., Heaton, R. K., Atkinson, J. H., et al. (2007). Neurocognitive effects of methamphetamine: a critical review and meta-analysis. *Neuropsychol Rev, 17*(3), 275-297.

Sekine, Y., Ouchi, Y., Takei, N., Yoshikawa, E., Nakamura, K., Futatsubashi, M., et al. (2006). Brain serotonin transporter density and aggression in abstinent methamphetamine abusers. *Arch Gen Psychiatry, 63*(1), 90-100.

Siegal, D., Erickson, J., Varoqui, H., Ang, L., Kalasinsky, K. S., Peretti, F. J., et al. (2004). Brain vesicular acetylcholine transporter in human users of drugs of abuse. *Synapse, 52*(4), 223-232.

Siegel, J. A., Benice, T. S., Van Meer, P., Park, B. S., & Raber, J. (2011). Acetylcholine receptor and behavioral deficits in mice lacking apolipoprotein E. *Neurobiol Aging, 32*, 75-84.

Siegel, J. A., Craytor, M. J., & Raber, J. (2010). Long-term effects of methamphetamine exposure on cognitive function and muscarinic acetylcholine receptor levels in mice. *Behav Pharmacol, 21*(7), 602-614.

Siegel, J. A., Park, B. S., & Raber, J. (2011). Long-term effects of neonatal methamphetamine exposure on cognitive function in adolescent mice. *Behav Brain Res, 219*(1), 159-164.

Silver, R. B., Mackins, C. J., Smith, N. C., Koritchneva, I. L., Lefkowitz, K., Lovenberg, T. W., et al. (2001). Coupling of histamine H3 receptors to neuronal Na+/H+ exchange: a novel protective mechanism in myocardial ischemia. *Proc Natl Acad Sci U S A, 98*(5), 2855-2859.

Smith, L. M., Lagasse, L. L., Derauf, C., Grant, P., Shah, R., Arria, A., et al. (2008). Prenatal methamphetamine use and neonatal neurobehavioral outcome. *Neurotoxicol Teratol, 30*(1), 20-28.

Smith, L. M., Lagasse, L. L., Derauf, C., Newman, E., Shah, R., Haning, W., et al. (2011). Motor and cognitive outcomes through three years of age in children exposed to prenatal methamphetamine. *Neurotoxicol Teratol, 33*(1), 176-184.

Sowell, E. R., Leow, A. D., Bookheimer, S. Y., Smith, L. M., O'Connor, M. J., Kan, E., et al. (2010). Differentiating Prenatal Exposure to Methamphetamine and Alcohol versus Alcohol and Not Methamphetamine using Tensor-Based Brain Morphometry and Discriminant Analysis. *J Neurosci, 30*(11), 3876-3885.

Steckler, T., & Holsboer, F. (2001). Interaction between the cholinergic system and CRH in the modulation of spatial discrimination learning in mice. *Brain Res, 906*(1-2), 46-59.

Struthers, J. M., & Hansen, R. L. (1992). Visual recognition memory in drug-exposed infants. *J Dev Behav Pediatr, 13*(2), 108-111.

Subramanian, N., Whitmore, W. L., Seidler, F. J., & Slotkin, T. A. (1981). Ontogeny of histaminergic neurotransmission in the rat brain: concomitant development of neuronal histamine, H-1 receptors, and H-1 receptor-mediated stimulation of phospholipid turnover. *J Neurochem, 36*(3), 1137-1141.

Sulzer, D., Sonders, M. S., Poulsen, N. W., & Galli, A. (2005). Mechanisms of neurotransmitter release by amphetamines: a review. *Prog Neurobiol, 75*(6), 406-433.

Taguchi, K., Atobe, J., Kato, M., Chuma, T., Chikuma, T., Shigenaga, T., et al. (1998). The effect of methamphetamine on the release of acetylcholine in the rat striatum. *Eur J Pharmacol, 360*(2-3), 131-137.

Terplan, M., Smith, E. J., Kozloski, M. J., & Pollack, H. A. (2009). Methamphetamine use among pregnant women. *Obstet Gynecol, 113*(6), 1285-1291.

Thal, L. J., Gilbertson, E., Armstrong, D. M., & Gage, F. H. (1992). Development of the basal forebrain cholinergic system: phenotype expression prior to target innervation. *Neurobiol Aging, 13*(1), 67-72.

Thiel, C. M. (2003). Cholinergic modulation of learning and memory in the human brain as detected with functional neuroimaging. *Neurobiol Learn Mem, 80*(3), 234-244.

Thompson, P. M., Hayashi, K. M., Simon, S. L., Geaga, J. A., Hong, M. S., Sui, Y., et al. (2004). Structural abnormalities in the brains of human subjects who use methamphetamine. *J Neurosci, 24*(26), 6028-6036.

Tran, V. T., Freeman, A. D., Chang, R. S., & Snyder, S. H. (1980). Ontogenetic development of histamine H1-receptor binding in rat brain. *J Neurochem, 34*(6), 1609-1613.

Trulson, M. E., Cannon, M. S., Faegg, T. S., & Raese, J. D. (1987). Tyrosine hydroxylase immunochemistry and quantitative light microscopic studies of the mesolimbic dopamine system in rat brain: effects of chronic methamphetamine administration. *Brain Res Bull, 18*(2), 269-277.

Uveges, A. J., Kowal, D., Zhang, Y., Spangler, T. B., Dunlop, J., Semus, S., et al. (2002). The role of transmembrane helix 5 in agonist binding to the human H3 receptor. *J Pharmacol Exp Ther, 301*(2), 451-458.

van Hest, A., Stroet, J., van Haaren, F., & Feenstra, M. (1990). Scopolamine differentially disrupts the behavior of male and female Wistar rats in a delayed nonmatching to position procedure. *Pharmacol Biochem Behav, 35*(4), 903-909.

Vanhala, A., Yamatodani, A., & Panula, P. (1994). Distribution of histamine-, 5-hydroxytryptamine-, and tyrosine hydroxylase-immunoreactive neurons and nerve fibers in developing rat brain. *J Comp Neurol, 347*(1), 101-114.

Vaucher, E., Reymond, I., Najaffe, R., Kar, S., Quirion, R., Miller, M. M., et al. (2002). Estrogen effects on object memory and cholinergic receptors in young and old female mice. *Neurobiol Aging, 23*(1), 87-95.

Volkow, N. D., Chang, L., Wang, G. J., Fowler, J. S., Franceschi, D., Sedler, M., et al. (2001). Loss of dopamine transporters in methamphetamine abusers recovers with protracted abstinence. *J Neurosci, 21*(23), 9414-9418.

Vorhees, C. V., Inman-Wood, S. L., Morford, L. L., Broening, H. W., Fukumura, M., & Moran, M. S. (2000). Adult learning deficits after neonatal exposure to D-methamphetamine: selective effects on spatial navigation and memory. *J Neurosci, 20*(12), 4732-4739.

Vorhees, C. V., Skelton, M. R., & Williams, M. T. (2007). Age-dependent effects of neonatal methamphetamine exposure on spatial learning. *Behav Pharmacol, 18*(5-6), 549-562.

Voytko, M. L., Olton, D. S., Richardson, R. T., Gorman, L. K., Tobin, J. R., & Price, D. L. (1994). Basal forebrain lesions in monkeys disrupt attention but not learning and memory. *J Neurosci, 14*(1), 167-186.

Wallace, T. L., Gudelsky, G. A., & Vorhees, C. V. (1999). Methamphetamine-induced neurotoxicity alters locomotor activity, stereotypic behavior, and stimulated dopamine release in the rat. *J Neurosci, 19*(20), 9141-9148.

Watanabe, T., & Yanai, K. (2001). Studies on functional roles of the histaminergic neuron system by using pharmacological agents, knockout mice and positron emission tomography. *Tohoku J Exp Med, 195*(4), 197-217.

Watson, M., Roeske, W. R., & Yamamura, H. I. (1986). [3H]pirenzepine and (-)-[3H]quinuclidinyl benzilate binding to rat cerebral cortical and cardiac muscarinic cholinergic sites. II. Characterization and regulation of antagonist binding to putative muscarinic subtypes. *J Pharmacol Exp Ther, 237*(2), 419-427.

West, M. J., Slomianka, L., & Gundersen, H. J. (1991). Unbiased stereological estimation of the total number of neurons in the subdivisions of the rat hippocampus using the optical fractionator. *Anat Rec, 231*(4), 482-497.

Whiteaker, P., Jimenez, M., McIntosh, J. M., Collins, A. C., & Marks, M. J. (2000). Identification of a novel nicotinic binding site in mouse brain using [(125)I]-epibatidine. *Br J Pharmacol, 131*(4), 729-739.

Wieland, K., Bongers, G., Yamamoto, Y., Hashimoto, T., Yamatodani, A., Menge, W. M., et al. (2001). Constitutive activity of histamine h(3) receptors stably expressed in SK-N-MC cells: display of agonism and inverse agonism by H(3) antagonists. *J Pharmacol Exp Ther, 299*(3), 908-914.

Williams, M. T., Blankenmeyer, T. L., Schaefer, T. L., Brown, C. A., Gudelsky, G. A., & Vorhees, C. V. (2003). Long-term effects of neonatal methamphetamine exposure in rats on spatial learning in the Barnes maze and on cliff avoidance, corticosterone release, and neurotoxicity in adulthood. *Brain Res Dev Brain Res, 147*(1-2), 163-175.

Winzer-Serhan, U. H. (2008). Long-term consequences of maternal smoking and developmental chronic nicotine exposure. *Front Biosci, 13*, 636-649.

Young, J. W., Crawford, N., Kelly, J. S., Kerr, L. E., Marston, H. M., Spratt, C., et al. (2007). Impaired attention is central to the cognitive deficits observed in alpha 7 deficient mice. *Eur Neuropsychopharmacol, 17*(2), 145-155.

Young, J. W., Finlayson, K., Spratt, C., Marston, H. M., Crawford, N., Kelly, J. S., et al. (2004). Nicotine improves sustained attention in mice: evidence for involvement of the alpha7 nicotinic acetylcholine receptor. *Neuropsychopharmacology, 29*(5), 891-900.

Zaborszky, L., Carlsen, J., Brashear, H. R., & Heimer, L. (1986). Cholinergic and GABAergic afferents to the olfactory bulb in the rat with special emphasis on the projection neurons in the nucleus of the horizontal limb of the diagonal band. *J Comp Neurol, 243*(4), 488-509.

Zahalka, E. A., Seidler, F. J., Lappi, S. E., Yanai, J., & Slotkin, T. A. (1993). Differential development of cholinergic nerve terminal markers in rat brain regions: implications for nerve terminal density, impulse activity and specific gene expression. *Brain Res, 601*(1-2), 221-229.

Zhu, J. P., Xu, W., & Angulo, J. A. (2006). Methamphetamine-induced cell death: selective vulnerability in neuronal subpopulations of the striatum in mice. *Neuroscience, 140*(2), 607-622.

Zule, W. A., Costenbader, E. C., Meyer, W. J., Jr., & Wechsberg, W. M. (2007). Methamphetamine use and risky sexual behaviors during heterosexual encounters. *Sex Transm Dis, 34*(9), 689-694.

In: Methamphetamines
Editors: J. Ornoy and X. He

ISBN: 978-1-62100-244-4

Chapter 2

WHAT CAN RODENT ACTIVITY TELL US ABOUT METHAMPHETAMINE ABUSE?

Andrew S. Sage and Dennis K. Miller*

Department of Psychological Sciences, Center for Translational Neuroscience, and Bond Life Science Center, University of Missouri, Columbia MO, US

ABSTRACT

Many abused drugs--including methamphetamine--produce a transient and dose-dependent change in locomotor behavior in rodents. Investigators can design experiments where methamphetamine is administered to rodents and locomotor behavior is observed, measured and analyzed, and many researchers have used this behavioral model to investigate the biological basis of methamphetamine's pharmacological activities. Moreover, several theories have been proposed to link locomotor activity findings in rodents to drug abuse and dependence in humans. This paper provides an overview of the theoretical basis of locomotor behavior as a model of human drug abuse and dependence, a critical comment on the methodological variables to be manipulated in a methamphetamine locomotor activity study, and a review of findings on the impact of multiple biological targets on methamphetamine-induced changes in locomotor behavior.

* Correspondence: Dennis K. Miller, Department of Psychological Sciences, University of Missouri, McAlester Hall, Columbia MO, 65210, USA. Tel: 573-884-8141, E-mail: millerden@missouri.edu.

INTRODUCTION

Addiction to psychostimulants, most notably methamphetamine and cocaine, is a pervasive and costly public health concern. Not only does methamphetamine use contribute to crime by adding to the number of incarcerated persons in state and federal correctional institutions and impose burdens on public and private health care sectors, it also has direct consequences on the lives of family members and communities at large (Hunt, 2006; U.S.DoJ, 2010). The prevalence of amphetamines has increased dramatically over the past twenty years: Between 1993 and 2007 the seizure of illicit amphetamines rose globally from 7 to 52 metric tons--an increase of 743% (U.N.O.D.C., 2009). This trend suggests that amphetamine abuse is an increasingly-important global issue.

While studying the after-effects of methamphetamine use is an option for investigating addiction in humans, animal models provide more practical empirical approaches to understanding both the acute and long-term effects of methamphetamine use. Animal models are particularly effective to characterize methamphetamine use over time (i.e., acute to repeated drug use) and to understand methamphetamine's mechanisms of action through the use of pharmacological and genetic manipulations. Researchers can administer methamphetamine and an experimental drug that acts at the same putative receptors as methamphetamine. Subsequent changes in behavior (e.g., responding on a lever or locomotor activity) can be measured in the presence and absence of the experimental drug and with acute or repeated methamphetamine treatment. Similarly, transgenic rodent lines can be generated to "knock-out" a specific protein to elucidate its role in methamphetamine's effects. These approaches have allowed researchers to understand the mechanisms involved in methamphetamine abuse and dependence.

Many abused drugs--including methamphetamine--derive their positively-reinforcing effects, at least in part, *via* activation of the mesolimbic dopamine pathway (Robinson & Berridge, 1993, 2000, 2001; Wise, 1998, 2002), dopamine-releasing neurons that project from the ventral tegmental area to the nucleus accumbens. Within the nucleus accumbens, methamphetamine blocks the activity of the vesicular monoamine transporter, a protein that normally sequesters dopamine into vesicular storage units, resulting in intraneuronal pools of "free" dopamine. Methamphetamine then induces the release of this dopamine into the extraneuronal space by reversing the activity of the dopamine transporter, a protein that normally shuttles dopamine from the extraneuronal space back into the neuron. Once outside the neuron, the dopamine binds to dopamine receptors. (A more thorough review of this process is presented in this volume in the chapter by Davis, Sage and Miller.). Methamphetamine's ability to suddenly and profoundly increase extracellular dopamine content is significant because this elevation is believed to contribute to stimulus salience and the development of drug craving that can follow repeated drug use (Robinson & Berridge, 1993). A stimulus (e.g. novelty, food, and methamphetamine) that induces dopamine release is perceived as rewarding and facilitates future stimulus recall and wanting the stimulus. In addition to its role on stimulus salience and craving, dopamine plays a critical role in the initiation of motor behavior and has been suggested to be an underlying factor in the locomotor activating properties common to all stimulants (Wise & Bozarth, 1987). However, individual differences in the response to drugs may be an important factor mediating the initiation and continuation of drug use (Bardo et al., 1996).

Animal models of genetically- or pharmacologically-manipulated proteins are extremely important to understand methamphetamine's mechanism of action. But, these models provide little benefit without dependent measures to quantify their effects on behavior. One example of animal behavior, crucial to our current understanding of methamphetamine's mechanisms of action, is locomotor activity. In the locomotor activity procedure, an animal, typically a rat or mouse, is allowed to freely traverse a large arena, called an open field. Locomotor behavior (e.g. the total distance travelled in centimeters or the number of instances of a specific type of behavior) can be measured and analyzed statistically. Numerous studies have shown that methamphetamine injection produces a marked change in locomotor activity, relative to the activity observed before drug injection or relative to a control group of animals treated with placebo (e.g. saline vehicle). Once the effect of methamphetamine on locomotor activity, within a specific dose range and over a specific period of time (e.g., acute versus repeated methamphetamine treatment) is determined, the effect of an experimental manipulation (e.g. receptor antagonism or genetic alteration) can be determined. Locomotor activity can be used to study both acute and repeated exposure to methamphetamine. With repeated methamphetamine treatment, a dynamic pattern of behavior develops where the locomotor response increases—becomes sensitized—even though the methamphetamine dose remains constant. Sensitization to methamphetamine-induced hyperactivity provides an animal model of the transition from "first-time user" (i.e., acute treatment) to "the addicted brain" (i.e., repeated treatment resulting in locomotor sensitization).

Animal models, including locomotor activity, are useful to the researcher because they provide the ability to test hypotheses and models of drug addiction derived from human patient experiences that cannot be tested empirically in humans. For example, drug-naïve rodents can be repeatedly administered methamphetamine, restricted in their access to methamphetamine to induce withdrawal symptoms, and then tested for their response to a later methamphetamine challenge. This is a protocol that could not be conducted empirically with human participants. Moreover, this protocol could examine the brain at the molecular level (e.g., levels of a specific protein) at different points during the protocol (e.g., before and after withdrawal).

Acute Methamphetamine Treatment

Most experiments that examine the effect of methamphetamine on locomotor behavior in rodents determine the impact after acute or sub-acute drug treatment. Typically, over the course of a short-period (e.g. 1 – 8 hours) the rodent receives a single or multiple (e.g., 2 – 4) methamphetamine treatments. This section describes variables and controls in the design of this type of short-term (acute) locomotor activity experiment.

There are several paradigms that can be used to quantify locomotor activity—circadian locomotor activity, activity wheels, locomotor activity in response to novelty, and open field test of exploratory activity. The most common paradigm used to measure locomotor activity is the open field design. Open field is a global measure of locomotor behavior generally, and exploratory behavior, specifically. In the typical open field procedure, a rat or mouse is placed into the center of a large arena (the open field) and behavior is measured. Figure 1 presents the open field activity monitor (Med Associates; Georgia, VT) used in our laboratory. The open field consists of a transparent (Plexiglas) box that is lined with intersecting banks of infrared sensors connected to a computer that records sensor-beam breaks in the x-, y-, and z-axis planes. An activity monitor can be visualized as a three-dimensional grid with a spatial resolution defined by the number of sensors on each axis. Recorded breaks can be analyzed alone or can be translated into distance traveled (e.g., centimeters) for analysis. Moreover, computer software, such as that prepared by Med Associates, can analyze breaks for stereotypy (a movement performed repeatedly, such as rocking back-and-forth), rotational behavior, and time in one part of the open field over other parts (e.g., time in the center versus the perimeter as a model of anxiety).

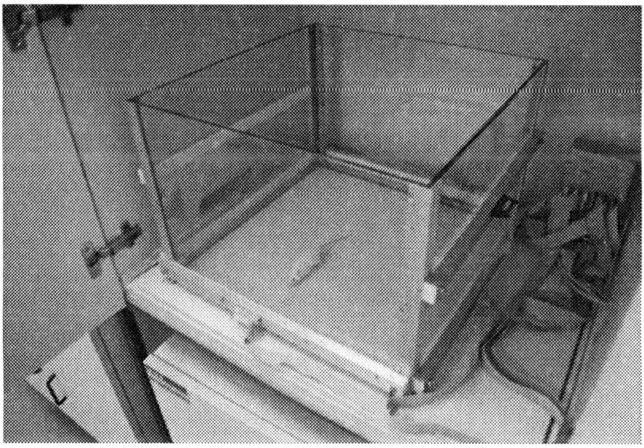

Figure 1. Locomotor Activity Monitor (Med Associates; Georgia, VT) with male CD-1 mouse. Two sets of infrared photo beams, perpendicularly aligned, provide *x*- and *y*-plane coverage. A single set of infrared photo beams running along the midline of the left and right sides provides *z*-plane coverage and can quantify rearing and climbing behaviors. In the upper-right of the photograph is an interface to a computer that can compute the number of beam breaks into dependent measures (e.g., distance traveled in centimeters or instances of stereotypy).

Any of the dependent measures (e.g., distance traveled or stereotypy) can be summed into as many discrete intervals (e.g. 5, 10, or 20 min) as are necessary to account for the locomotor activity session. Interval size is based on the overall session duration and the expected time course of the drug's effects (e.g. an increase and decrease in behavior within minutes compared to a prolonged drug change over several hours). For example, if locomotor activity is measured for 30 minutes, summing into 10-minute intervals would produce only three data points, and may not be informative of the drug's time course. A cost-benefit ratio of temporal resolution versus data set size may be a consideration. An important variable to account for when planning the parameters of a locomotor activity study is to determine the time course of drug effect through its kinetic profile. As an example, if Drug X administration yields peak blood/brain levels 30 minutes after treatment, and has a half-life of two hours; measuring activity only during a 30-minute post-administration period would yield only part of the drug's effects on locomotor behavior.

The open field paradigm is frequently used for between-group designs, but may also be used for within-subjects designs. A between-group design involves comparisons between two or more groups, where at least one group serves as a control (e.g. placebo treatment) and the other groups are experimental manipulation (e.g., methamphetamine treatments). A within-subjects design involves comparing a single group before and after treatment. For example, a single group's baseline locomotor activity in response to vehicle injection is measured and then methamphetamine is administered subsequently. Activity during vehicle and methamphetamine treatment can then be compared. Drug-induced hyper- or hypo-locomotor activity can be qualified as either a positive or negative change, respectively, relative to control.

Habituation sessions provide the necessary baseline against which the experimental group can be contrasted. If an experimental manipulation is expected to produce hyperactivity, as methamphetamine treatment does, it is important to habituate all animals to the activity monitors before introducing the drug injection regimen. Habituation will reduce the potential for confounds such as novelty-induced freezing and exploratory behaviors. However, habituation might not be preferred if the drug is predicted to reduce locomotor activity on its own (e.g., alcohol or benzodiazepines) because habituated animals will already show decreased locomotion.

Once the methamphetamine dose-response curve is determined, the impact of another variable, such as a receptor antagonist, can be investigated. For example, Li and colleagues (2006), conducted a locomotor activity study examining the effects of valproic acid, an anti-convulsant that modulates GABA neurotransmission, on methamphetamine (2 mg/kg)-induced hyper-activity in mice. The protocol was designed around the prediction that valproic acid's maximal therapeutic effects were likely to be observed 30 - 120 minutes post-injection in mice. Mice were habituated to the locomotor activity monitor for 15 minutes prior to any drug injection, and valproic acid was given 30 minutes prior to methamphetamine administration. Li determined the impact of acute (i.e., single) drug treatment and the effect of repeated (once-daily for 7 days) drug treatments on the development and expression of locomotor sensitization to psychostimulants (e.g. cocaine and methamphetamine).

Byrnes-Blake and colleagues (2003), present a locomotor protocol using male Sprague-Dawley rats. Rats were habituated to the testing environment for a minimum of three hours per day, for four to six days, prior to beginning the experiment. Multiple methamphetamine doses (0.3, 1, and 3 mg/kg) were examined and this dose range was selected because it had previously been shown to reliably produce differences in distance traveled without inducing self-mutilation (a form of stereotypy) or death. Methamphetamine injections were given 30 minutes prior to the experimental manipulation (an anti-methamphetamine antibody) because previous data from their lab indicated that methamphetamine and its metabolite (amphetamine) approach maximum concentration at this time-point. Three dependent variables—distance traveled, number of rearing events, and time spent moving—were measured and analyzed.

Experiment on the Effect of Methamphetamine on Locomotor Activity in Mice

Figures 2 and 3 present the findings from an experiment in our laboratory to determine the effect of a range (0.158 – 5 mg/kg) of methamphetamine doses on locomotor activity in mice after a single administration. A between-groups design was used where different groups of mice received the different methamphetamine doses or control (0 mg/kg methamphetamine, saline vehicle) treatment. Distance traveled (in centimeters) was the dependent variable.

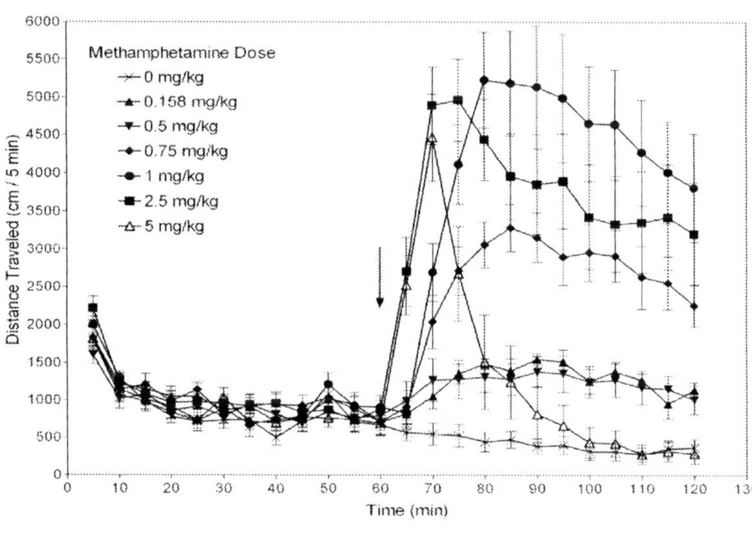

Figure 2. Methamphetamine changes locomotor activity following a single administration to mice. Male CD-1 mice were placed in an automated activity monitor for 60 minutes, administered (i.p.) methamphetamine (0, 0.158 – 5 mg/kg; designated by the arrow) and returned to the monitor for 60 minutes. Data represent mean (±S.E.M.) distance traveled in 5-minute intervals. These data, summed across the 60-min post-injection period, are presented in Figure 3.

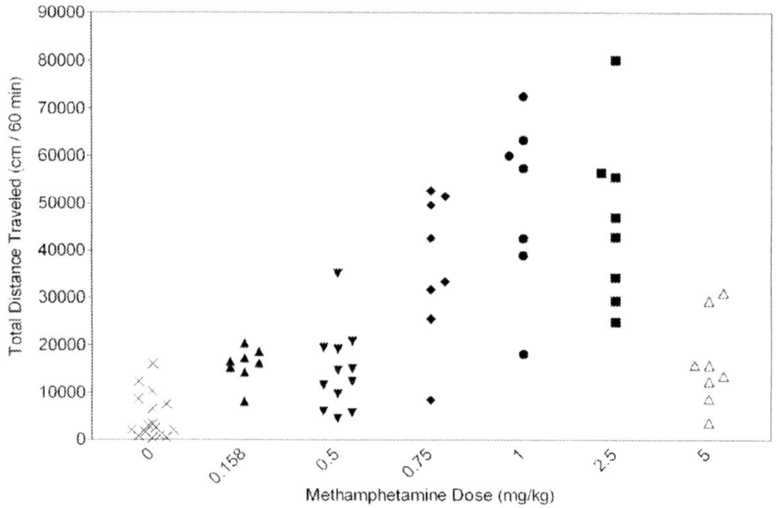

Figure 3. Male CD-1 mice were placed in an automated activity monitor for 60 minutes, administered (i.p.) methamphetamine (0, 0.158 – 5 mg/kg) and returned to the monitor for 60 minutes. Data points represent distance traveled during the 60-minute interval after injection for individual mice. These data, presented across the 60-minute post-injection session in 5-min intervals, are also depicted in Figure 2.

Male CD-1 mice, weighing ~25 g, were acclimated to the animal colony for one to two weeks upon arrival to the laboratory. For two consecutive days the mice were habituated to the activity monitors. On these days mice were handled by the experimenter, weighed, and placed in the activity monitor (Figure 1) for 30-60 minutes. On the following day, mice were returned to the activity monitor for a 60-minute rehabituation trial followed by methamphetamine (0.158 – 5 mg/kg) or saline injection (i.p.). Mice remained in the monitor for 60 minutes after injection.

Figure 2 shows the results of the methamphetamine dose-response test. The time-course of drug effects is a presentation of mean distance traveled (in centimeters) in 5-minute intervals. The downward-facing arrow indicates methamphetamine administration. As the methamphetamine dose increases from saline (0 mg/kg) through 1 mg/kg so too does the locomotor response. However, at the 2.5 mg/kg dose, a slight decrease in activity, relative to the 1 mg/kg dose group, is observed. When the methamphetamine dose is increased to 5 mg/kg, a steep decline in total distance traveled beginning within the first 15 minutes post-injection is observed. This behavioral shift reflects the transition of behavioral activation from locomotor to stereotypic behavior (which was not analyzed).

Figure 3 presents the data depicted in Figure 2 in a different format. For Figure 3 the total distance traveled in each 5-minute interval over the 60 minute post-injection period, were summed to a single data point (i.e., the area under the curves from Figure 2). The data follow the same basic trend of increasing activity from the 0.158 through the 1 mg/kg dose with a decline in activity at the 2.5 and 5.0 mg/kg doses. In the literature, locomotor activity data are typically presented as the mean or median with "error bars" reflecting standard error or standard deviation of the mean. (Figure 2 presents the time-course data as mean and standard error.) Figure 3 presents the data as a scatter plot where data from each mouse is presented. There is great variability in the locomotor response among mice that received the same methamphetamine dose. This variability is typical for the locomotor activity procedure and an investigator may need a relatively-large number of subjects in each group to determine statistically-significant differences. However, the variability parallels the individual differences in drug responding observed in human subjects (Comings & Blum, 2000; Haile, Kosten & Kosten, 2009). Researchers can use this observed variability to investigate differences between "high responders" and "low responders": A large group of mice can be tested with methamphetamine and the upper and lower percentiles or a median split can be used to generate separate groups (Bevins & Peterson, 2004).

Factors for the Design and Conduct of Locomotor Experiments

The experiment presented in Figures 2 and 3 reflects a single methamphetamine injection to the mice. An alternative procedure is to administer several (e.g., 2 – 4 administrations) methamphetamine doses over short (e.g., 2 hour) intervals during a single day. This procedure can be used to model human methamphetamine use where the user might administer the drug at intervals over the course of several hours (Dluzen & Liu, 2008). In rodents, sporadic administration may produce greater stereotypy than a single methamphetamine injection. Furthermore, repeated administration of higher methamphetamine doses (e.g., $\geq \sim 2$ mg/kg) may be used to study methamphetamine neurotoxicity. For example, a decrease in proteins involved in dopamine synthesis and storage (e.g., tyrosine hydroxylase or the vesicular monoamine transporter) may be observed (Steinkellner et al., 2011).

Table 1. Examples of locomotor activity studies in mice

Mouse Strain	Parameters & Dose	Relevant Findings
C57BL/6J	Two 5-hr habituation trials to apparatus; 2-5 mg/kg methamphetamine (s.c.); 5 hr test in 20-minute intervals.	Dobbs et al (2008) reported methamphetamine dose-dependently increases extracellular dopamine and acetylcholine levels.
C57BL/6J	Habituation for 3-8 days to the home cage, which also served as the testing apparatus; 2-4 mg/kg methamphetamine (i.p.); 150-minute test in 15-minute intervals, with 60 minute pretest and 90 minute post drug treatment.	Zombeck et al (2009 & 2010) reported adolescent (30-35 days old) mice are less sensitive to methamphetamine's locomotor-activating properties than adult (69-74 days old) mice.
C57BL/6J	No habituation, 5 mg/kg methamphetamine (i.p.) administered 1 or 3 times in 2-hr intervals; mice tested in T-maze.	Glickstein and Schmauss (2004a & 2004b) reported one methamphetamine treatment increases locomotor activity, while multiple produce orofacial stereotypy. The D2 dopamine receptor is critical for the acute response to methamphetamine and for recovery of spatial working memory deficits.
DBA/2J	Habituation to the behavioral test room for 45-60 minutes, but not the apparatus; 2 mg/kg methamphetamine (i.p.); 30 minute test in 5-minute intervals.	Kamens and Phillips (2008) reported the 2 mg/kg methamphetamine dose produces robust locomotor activity.
ddY	Two 60-minute habituation trials; 2 mg/kg methamphetamine (s.c.); 120 minute test in 15-minute intervals.	Nakagawa et al (2005) reported methamphetamine-induced locomotor activity (2 mg/kg) is not affected by GLT-1 activation.

Mouse Strain	Parameters & Dose	Relevant Findings
ddY	60-minute habituation immediately prior to drug administration; 0.64-10 mg/kg methamphetamine (i.p.); 4-hr test with 10 behavioral ratings made within 90 seconds, each 15-minute interval.	Yamanaka et al (1983) reported a biphasic dose-response curve on locomotor activity, with stereotypy at higher (≥ 5 mg/kg) doses.
ddY	30-minute habituation immediately prior to drug administration; 1-2 mg/kg methamphetamine (i.p.); 60-minute test in 5-minute intervals.	Ago et al (2009) reported adrenalectomy or glucocorticoid receptor antagonism attenuates methamphetamine-induced hyperactivity

Regarding an investigation of methamphetamine, there are a number of experimental parameters that can be manipulated to study its effects on locomotor behavior. Table 1 provides an overview and summary of a variety of parameters that have been used in different reports using mice. Within the table is a list of mouse strains, experimental parameters, methamphetamine doses, and relevant experimental findings *via* the procedures used. Included in the table are both low-dose acute (i.e., less than 2 mg/kg, methamphetamine) and repeated high-dose (i.e., more than one treatment of greater than 5 mg/kg methamphetamine) methamphetamine treatments.

Krasonova and colleagues (2007) provide a detailed explanation of open field novelty-induced locomotor activity and a neurological test battery, which can serve as an animal model of a clinical neurological examination. The paper by Krasnova also provides a narrative of high-performance liquid chromatography, histology, microarray hybridization with its statistical analysis, and quantitative reverse transcriptase polymerase chain reaction techniques that may alert the reader to a variety of possible *in vitro* measures that may supplement activity findings.

The benefits of using locomotor activity to study methamphetamine are numerous. First, the behavioral response is dose- and time-dependent (Figures 2 and 3), which allows for a true pharmacological analysis where the dose-response curve could be "shifted" by another variable (e.g., receptor antagonist or as a consequence of conditioning). Second, the paradigm provides a global measure of behavior that models "first-time drug use". Acute locomotor activity provides a necessary contrast for other animal models of drug addiction (such as sensitization, *vide infra*), permitting inquiry of the possible differences between initial drug use and use by an "addict". By contrasting the acute response to the response after repeated methamphetamine treatment, investigators can better understand changes occurring as a result of recurrent drug exposure. This may help address the question, "What are the behavioral differences, if any, between first-time and addicted drug users?". A third benefit of locomotor activity is that it can be used as a tool for researchers to investigate the different neurotransmitters and signaling pathways involved in methamphetamine's mechanism of action. Through the use of pharmacological agents (e.g., receptor antagonists), a greater understanding of methamphetamine in the brain and body can be obtained. This approach has helped to identify proteins that are (and are not) necessary for methamphetamine-induced behavioral activation (Table 2) as well as the cortical and sub-cortical circuits that may be influenced by repeated drug use. A fourth advantage of the procedure is that it may provide insight into the individual succeptibility and potential biological bases of vulnerability to drug addiction (Comings & Blum, 2000; Bevins & Peterson, 2004; Haile et al., 2009). For example, it may be possible to correlate genotypic data with methamphetamine-induced locomotor activity. It might be found that the few rodents who fail to respond to methamphetamine or those that do, but do so to a much lesser degree, share or commonly lack a unique biomarker (e.g., a receptor subtype). Possible links between specific biomarkers and the psychomotor stimulating effects of methamphetamine could then be determined. A final benefit is simplicity. The paradigm is relatively easy to use, it can be fully automated, and it can be used for rats or mice. Locomotor activity can be an incredibly efficient, reliable, and flexible behavioral measure.

Despite the many useful applications of acute locomotor activity, there are a few disadvantages. First, due to the exploratory nature of open field, the apparatus will need to be set up in low- or no-light conditions, because rodents typically explore in the dark, and may display freezing behaviors in bright-light conditions. Second, novelty plays an excitatory role in the exploratory behavior of mice and rats, and it is often necessary to provide pre-treatment trials to habituate rodents to the open field. Habituation trials typically involve *at least* one or two 30 - 60 minute exposures to the training apparatus in the days leading up to measuring locomotor activity. A third disadvantage of the locomotor activity procedure is that it does not provide a direct measure of drug-taking behavior, as observed with the self-administration procedure. In the locomotor activity procedure the amount of methamphetamine administered and when it is delivered is controlled by the investigator, and not the rodent, as it is in the self-administration procedure (Pickens & Thompson,

1968). Despite its limitations, psychological and biological theories suggest that locomotor activity can be used to study, indirectly, the reinforcing and reinforcing properties of methamphetamine (Robinson & Berridge, 1993, 2000, 2001; Wise & Bozarth, 1987).

Biological and Theoretical Basis of Locomotor Activity

Biologically-based theories of drug addiction have focused on dopamine's role (Robinson & Berridge, 1993, 2000; Bardo et al., 1996; *vide infra*) and the behavioral effects of methamphetamine are related to its ability to increase dopamine levels in brain (Fornai et al., 2009). Researchers have used the locomotor activity assay in rodents to investigate methamphetamine's mechanisms of action, and much research has focused on dopamine (Rubinstein et al., 1997; Kelly et al., 2008; Krasnova et al., 2009; Zombeck et al., 2009). However, other neuroactive ligands such as acetylcholine (Shimosato et al., 2001, 2003; Dobbs et al., 2008; Kamens & Phillips, 2008; Camarasa et al., 2009), cannabinoids (Ishiguro et al., 2010), histamine (Inoue et al., 1996; Toyota et al., 2003), serotonin (Ginawi et al., 2004, 2005; Picard et al., 2010), excitatory amino acids (glutamate; Nakagawa et al., 2005; Hagino et al., 2010), and sigma receptor ligands (Nguyen et al., 2005; Matsumoto et al., 2008; Rodvelt et al., 2011) have been investigated and shown to influence the effects of methamphetamine on locomotor behavior. Table 2 is an overview of the signaling systems that have been shown to play a role.

Drug addiction is a complex and multifaceted problem (for review, Thomas, 2006; Winger, Woods, & Hofmann, 2004). Historically-early theories considered addiction as a weakness of character ("moral theory") or as a medical issue for treatment ("disease theory"). In the twentieth century behavioral theories focused on either the positive ("reward theory") or negative ("dependence theory") reinforcing drug effects and were based on the pharmacological properties of depressants (e.g., alcohol and narcotics). Dependence theories posited that addicts are compelled to relieve the physical and/or psychological withdrawal symptoms that result when drug use is discontinued. However, these theories did not address the biological mechanisms responsible for these symptoms or consider the underlying motivations that may lead to exploratory drug use and initial drug experiences. Reward theories have attempted to explain a drug user's first experiences with a drug as curiosity, with subsequent use mediated by the subjective euphoric or pleasurable state induced by the initial drug experiences. Animal models, such as observation of antagonist-precipitated withdrawal, self-administration, and place conditioning have been used to support and reject the dependence and reward (and other) theories of drug addiction. Over the past quarter century other theories (e.g., the Psychomotor Stimulant and the Incentive-Sensitization theories) of drug addiction have been developed around the locomotor activity model.

Table 2. Signaling systems implicated in methamphetamine-induced locomotor activity in rats and mice

Signaling System	Rodent Species	Relevant Findings
Acetylcholine		
	CD-1 mice	Camarasa et al (2009) reported that repeated, but not acute nicotine exposure potentiates methamphetamine-induced locomotor activity, which was suppressed by nicotinic receptor antagonists (methyllcaconatine and DHβE).
	DBA/2J mice	Kamens and Phillips (2008) reported neuronal nicotinic receptors are involved in acute alcohol-induced, but not methamphetamine-induced, stimulation.
	C57BL/6J mice	Dobbs and colleagues (2008) reported methamphetamine-induced hyperactivity activity dose-dependently correlates with extrasynaptic acetylcholine, but not dopamine levels in the ventral tegmental area.
	ddY mice	Shimosato et al (2001) reported muscarinic receptor antagonists (scopolamine and trihexyphenidyl) facilitate methamphetamine-induced locomotor activity.
Cannabinoid		
	C57BL/6J mice	Ishiguro et al (2010) reported CB2 cannabinoid receptor antagonism (via AM-630) increases methamphetamine-induced locomotor activity
Dopamine		
	C57BL/6J mice	Kelly et al (2008) reported D2 dopamine receptor knock-out mice, relative to wild-type mice, showed a reduced locomotor response to methamphetamine and are more sensitive to D1 dopamine receptor antagonist (SCH-23390) effects on methamphetamine
	C57BL/6J mice	Rubinstein et al (1997) reported D4 dopamine receptor knock-out reduces spontaneous behavior, but increased methamphetamine-induced locomotor activity and increased dopamine synthesis and metabolites in dorsal striata, relative to wild-type mice.

Signaling System	Rodent Species	Relevant Findings
	BALB/c mice	Krasnova et al (2009) reported acute high dose methamphetamine treatment produces a long-lasting deficit in basal locomotor activity.
	C57BL/6J mice	Zombeck et al (2009) reported neurodevelopmental differences lead adolescent (30-35 days old) mice to be less sensitive to methamphetamine's locomotor activating properties than adult (69-74 days old) mice.
	C57BL mice	Kobayashi and Sano (2000) reported no methamphetamine-induced hyperactivity in tyrosine hydroxylase knock-out mice
GABA		
	Swiss Webster mice	Ungard et al (2009) reported the $GABA_A$ GABA receptor allosteric modulator ganaxolone does not prevent methamphetamine-induced hyperactivity.
Glucocorticoids		
	ddY mice	Ago et al (2009) reported glucocorticoid receptor antagonism or adrenalectomy attenuates methamphetamine-induced hyperactivity.
Glutamate		
	ddY mice	Nakagawa et al (2005) reported glutamate transporter activation (MS-153) does not affect methamphetamine-induced changes in locomotor behavior.
	C57BL mice	Hagino et al (2010) reported no effect of GluRε1 or GluRε4 glutamate receptor knock-out on methamphetamine-induced hyperactivity.
Histamine		
	C57BL/6J mice	Toyota et al (2003) reported H3 histamine receptor knock-out mice display reduced methamphetamine-induced hyperactivity, relative to wild-type mice
Norepinephrine		
	ICR mice	Okuyama et al (1997) Uzuki et al (2002) reported adrenoceptor antagonists (NRA0045 and NRA0161, respectively) decrease methamphetamine-induced hyperactivity

Table 2. Continued

Signaling System	Rodent Species	Relevant Findings
Opioid		
	ddY mice	Mori et al (2006) reported opioid receptor agonists (morphine and buprenorphine) diminish methamphetamine-induced stereotypy without affecting spontaneous activity.
Serotonin		
	Swiss Albino mice	Picard et al (2010) reported $5HT_{1A}$ serotonin receptor agonism (JB-788) dose-dependently attenuates methamphetamine-induced hyper activity.
	Swiss Albino mice	Ginawi et al (2004) reported $5\text{-}HT_{1B/1D}$ and $5\text{-}HT_{2C}$ serotonin receptor antagonism (methiothepin and mianserin, respectively) attenuates methamphetamine-induced hyperactivity. $5HT_{2A/2B}$ and $5\text{-}HT_3$ serotonin receptor antagonism (methysergide and ondansetron, respectively) potentiates methamphetamine-induced hyperactivity.
	Swiss Albino mice	Ginawi et al (2005) reported $5\text{-}HT_{1A}$ receptor antagonism (NAN-190) diminishes methamphetamine-induced hyperactivity.
	ICR mice	Yoo et al (2008, 2010) reported $5HT_3$ serotonin receptor antagonism (MDL-72222) attenuates methamphetamine-induced hyperactivity, an effect linked to GABA and DA activity.
Sigma		
	Sprague-Dawley rats	Rodvelt et al (2011) reported σ1 sigma receptor agonism/antagonism (SA 4503) both potentiates and inhibits methamphetamine-induced hyperactivity.
	Swiss Webster mice	Matsumoto et al (2008) reported σ1 sigma receptor antagonism (AC927) attenuates methamphetamine-induced hyperactivity.
	Swiss Webster mice	Nguyen et al (2005) reported σ_1 sigma receptor antagonism (BD1063 and BD1047) and antisense oligodeoxynucleotide-mediated down-regulation attenuates methamphetamine-induced hyperactivity.

Wise and Bozarth's Psychomotor Stimulant Theory of Addiction (1987) provides a theoretical basis for considering locomotor behavior in a model of drug addiction. Wise and Bozarth proposed that all drugs of abuse have psychomotor stimulant actions. There is a common biological mechanism (e.g., dopamine in the brain) for the production of psychomotor stimulant actions, and this biological mechanism overlaps with the mechanisms for positive reinforcement. More succinctly, all addictive drugs are positively reinforcing in that they produce behavioral activation (e.g. drug seeking) through a common biological mechanism. Methamphetamine is a prototype for this theory because it has dynamic locomotor-activating properties. Studying the effects of acute and repeated methamphetamine treatment in rodents on locomotion, with the aid of pharmacological and genetic manipulations, may elucidate the biological mechanisms underlying methamphetamine-induced behaviors, including positive reinforcement.

7There are two dopamine pathways—the mesolimbic from the ventral tegmental area to the nucleus accumbens and nigrostriatal from the substantia nigra to the basal ganglia—that are relevant to the Psychomotor Stimulant Theory of Addiction. From the standpoint that these dopamine pathways belong to a phylogenetically old system, conserved across mammalian species, Bardo (1996) has proposed that the dopamine system was likely conserved because it sub-serves behaviors vital to survival. For example, dopamine is proposed to be the principle neurotransmitter involved in locomotion, emotion, learning, and neuroendocrine modulation (Kobayashi & Sano, 2000). A role for the mesolimbic dopamine reward pathway in approach and investigatory behaviors (i.e., novelty seeking) has also been suggested (Bardo et al., 1996) Indeed, the mesolimbic dopamine pathway has been deemed a final common pathway for many natural rewards (e.g. novelty and food) as well as for alcohol, cocaine, and methamphetamine (Kamens & Phillips, 2008). The nigrostriatal pathway regulates cortical outputs essential for executing motor behaviors (Graybiel et al., 1994), largely through dopamine transmission. The vital role of dopamine in motor movements is highlighted in Parkinson's disease, which results from the degeneration of dopamine cell bodies (and their corresponding axons) in the nigrostriatal pathway (for review, Shadrina et al., 2010). In this dopamine-based framework, methamphetamine administration increases the activity of mesolimbic and nigrostriatal pathways, which leads to enhanced approach and investigatory behaviors, as well as enhanced execution of locomotor behaviors.

Bardo and colleagues (1996) proposed that drug addiction theories might be more easily conceptualized as either adaptive or exposure theories.

Exposure theories suggest that all mammals are susceptible, or "at risk", for developing drug addiction. The critical factor in determining which organism will and which will not develop addiction, is exposure to the drug. This idea can be related back to the reward theory, where the initial euphoric effects motivate subsequent use. Intuitively, if an organism never comes into contact with a drug, it cannot experience its subjective euphoric effects, and thus cannot develop drug addiction. However, this posits that drug exposure will inevitably promote future drug seeking tendencies, leading to addiction. In contrast to exposure theories, adaptive theories argue that exposure to a drug while necessary, is not sufficient to produce addiction. Rather, individual differences in the initial drug response may govern or even predict whether or not continued use will develop. One such adaptive theory is the Incentive-Sensitization Theory of Addiction proposed by Robinson and Berridge (1993, 2000, 2001).

Robinson and Berridge observed that with repeated administration, addictive drugs enhance dopamine neurotransmission in the midbrain (e.g., mesolimbic and nigrostriatal dopamine pathways). These neural changes could be conceptualized as Hebbian plasticity, or a strengthening of synaptic connections via sustained and synchronous neuronal firing (Kandel, Schwartz, & Jessell, 1995). As dopamine neurotransmission becomes enhanced, the psychological effects of the drug change: The user transitions from using the drug because he "likes" it to using the drug because he "craves" it. With further increases in dopamine neurotransmission the drug gains stimulus salience, or "importance". Stimulus salience may also be further enhanced by contextual cues associated with the drug (e.g., the sights, sounds and odors that occur before or with drug administration). As a drug is repeatedly administered in a particular environment, the drug's psychological effects may become increasingly associated with the contextual cues (Hall et al., 2008). Over time, presentation of the cues, even in the absence of drug, may induce drug "craving" and seeking behaviors. Additionally, the magnitude or extent of the drug "craving" and seeking behaviors may become sensitized over time. Behavioral sensitization may be responsible for the increased drug seeking behaviors (Vezina, 2004: Scibelli et al., 2011), even in the face of severe consequences, observed in human methamphetamine users (Tabibnia et al., 2011). Sensitization may also provide an explanation of the relapse to drug taking behavior observed in many struggling-to-abstain users: Relapse may be precipitated by exposure to contextual cues (e.g., a "drug house" or other users) associated with previous drug taking.

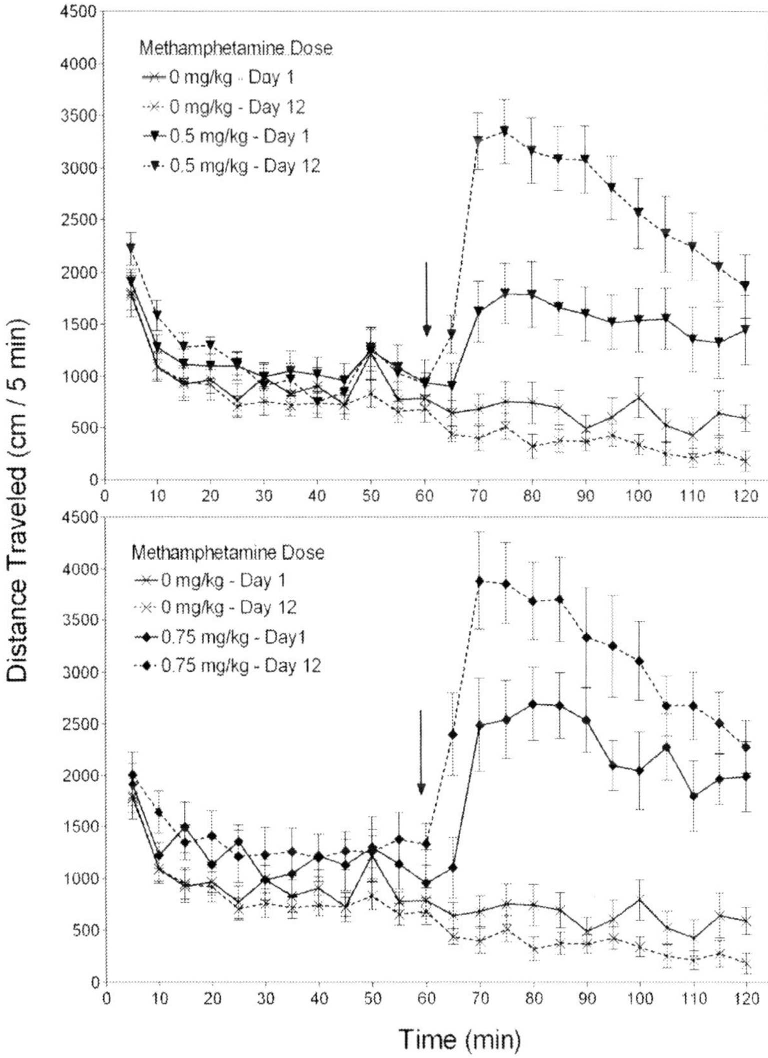

Figure 4. Sensitization develops to methamphetamine-induced hyperactivity in mice. For five consecutive days (Days 1 – 5), male CD-1 mice were placed in an automated activity monitor for 60 minutes and then injected (i.p.) with methamphetamine (0.158 [data not shown], 0.5 or 0.75 mg/kg) or saline (0 mg/kg) and returned to the monitor for 60 minutes. Downward-facing arrows indicate methamphetamine or saline injection. Rats were not tested on the next 6 days (Days 6 – 11) and were reintroduced to the experimental procedures on Day 12. Data represent mean (±S.E.M.) distance traveled in 5-minute intervals on Day 1 and Day 12. These data are also depicted in Figure 5 as the total distance traveled during the 60-minute post-injection period on Days 1 – 5 and 12.

Methamphetamine Sensitzation

Behavioral sensitization can be observed and measured in the locomotor activity model in rodents. Sensitization is an increase in the behavioral response with repeated treatment with the same drug dose. For example, if a mouse is administered 1 mg/kg methamphetamine once a day for five consecutive days, locomotor activity might increase from 5,000 cm/session following the first injection (compared to 1,000 cm/session for saline-treated mice) to 15,000 cm/session following the fifth injection. Thus, methamphetamine produced hyperactivity on the first injection (between-group comparison between methamphetamine- and saline-treated mice) and sensitization developed to this hyperactivity with repeated methamphetamine treatment (within-subjects comparison for methamphetamine-treated rats from the first to the fifth injection). Sensitization can be considered the opposite of tolerance, where the effect of a drug diminishes with repeated treatment.

The advantage of the behavioral sensitization model for drug abuse researchers is that it permits investigation of the development, persistence, and relapse of addiction. Measures of acute effects of methamphetamine on locomotor activity, as previously described, provide a picture of what happens when a drug is used for the first time. But, this may not be informative when trying to understand dependence and addiction, processes that occur with repeated methamphetamine treatment. In this regard, sensitization models the transitions from "drug-naïve" to "experienced drug user" and "liking" methamphetamine to "craving" methamphetamine, as proposed by Robinson and Berridge (1993, 2000, 2001). As such, the procedure might be used as a model to test therapeutic interventions that will be used in humans who have a long history of drug use. For example, our laboratory showed that lobeline, a botanical product that has potential as a methamphetamine pharmacotherapy, blocks the sensitization that develops after repeated cocaine treatment (Polston et al., 2006). These preclinical data suggest lobeline could have potential as a cocaine addiction pharmacotherapy.

Locomotor sensitization can be viewed from two temporal perspectives—initiation and expression. Studies investigating the initiation of sensitization to drug induced-hyperactivity explore variables that lead to, prevent, or otherwise alter the development and onset of drug sensitization. The expression of sensitization represents behaviors after the sensitized response is observed. While initiation studies look at variables that can be manipulated to reduce or prevent sensitization development, expression studies look at ways to reduce or alter the sensitized response once it has developed. Activating or inhibiting a biological target might block the initiation, the expression or both the initiation and expression of sensitization to methamphetamine. For example, to test the effect of Drug X on the initiation of sensitization to methamphetamine-induced hyperactivity, mice would receive Drug X and methamphetamine concurrently and repeatedly. Then, methamphetamine would be administered in the absence of Drug X. Did Drug X prevent the development of sensitization to methamphetamine or did it merely "mask" it from being observed? To test the effect of Drug Y on the expression of sensitization to methamphetamine-induced hyperactivity, mice would receive only methamphetamine repeatedly. Then, Drug Y and methamphetamine would be administered on the same session. Is the sensitized response still present or has it been affected by Drug Y?

Experiment on the Effect of Repeated Methamphetamine on Locomotor Activity in Mice

Figures 4, 5 and 6 present the findings from an experiment in our laboratory to determine the effect of a range (0.158 – 5 mg/kg) of methamphetamine doses on locomotor activity in mice after repeated administration. Similar to our earlier experiment (Figures 2 and 3), a between-groups design was used where different groups of mice received the different methamphetamine doses or control (0 mg/kg methamphetamine, saline vehicle) treatment; however, each mouse received the same drug treatment on each test day. Mice first received two habituation sessions. On the following day (Day 1) mice were placed in the monitor for 60 minutes, administered methamphetamine (0.158 – 5 mg/kg) or saline vehicle (0 mg/kg) and returned the chamber for 60 min. The procedure from Day 1 was repeated for four more days (Days 2 – 5). On Days 6 – 11 mice remained in the animal colony, and were not administered drug or placed in the activity monitors. However, on Day 12, mice were tested as they had been on Days 1 – 5.

Figure 4 depicts a sensitized response to methamphetamine by contrasting Day 1 to Day 12. On Day 1, both 0.5 and 0.75 mg/kg methamphetamine produced hyperactivity, relative to the rats administered only saline (0 mg/kg). (Data from mice administered 0.158 mg/kg methamphetamine are not presented in Figure 4.) On Day 12, the response to that same methamphetamine dose is greater (~10 - 75%) than it was on Day 1: Sensitization developed to the methamphetamine-induced hyperactivity. The methamphetamine doses used in this locomotor sensitization experiment are lower than the maximum doses used for the acute locomotor activity experiments (compare Figures 2 and 4). The premise of sensitization is that increased behavior is observed with repeated administration. If the acute response was maximal on Day 1, it would not have been possible to observe sensitization to the hyperactivity, an example of a "ceiling effect." The mice that received saline displayed a decrease (~5 - 50%) in their locomotor response from Day 1 to Day 12.

Figure 5 depicts the total distance traveled over the 60 minute post-injection period on Days 1 - 5 and 12. It is clear that sensitization does not develop to repeated saline administration. Rather, it results in a decrease in locomotor activity from Day 1 to Day 12. The 0.158 mg/kg methamphetamine dose produced hyperactivity on Day 1, relative to saline (0 mg/kg)-treated mice. However, while the hyperactivity persisted across Days 1 to 12, sensitization did not develop to this dose of methamphetamine. Robust hyperactivity was displayed on each day for mice that received 0.5 mg/kg methamphetamine. Sensitization developed to methamphetamine-induced hyperactivity by Day 4. For the mice administered the 0.75 mg/kg methamphetamine dose, hyperactivity was observed on each day, but sensitization, relative to Day 1, was only evident on Day 12. Furthermore, there was a decrease in methamphetamine-induced hyperactivity for this group on Days 2 and 3.

Recall that acute locomotor activity findings (e.g., Figure 3) and adaptive theories of addiction (e.g., Bardo et al., 1996) suggest that individual differences among subjects in their initial response to methamphetamine exist. Not surprisingly, individual variability is also present in the initiation of locomotor sensitization to methamphetamine, and this was evident in our experiment. Figure 6 shows the locomotor response to methamphetamine (0.75 mg/kg) for individual mice on Days 1 – 5 and 12. The total distance traveled over the 60-minute post-injection period on each day is represented by a symbol to show variability among mice. The lines "connect" the activity for each mouse across days. Note the lines labeled A, B and C in Figure 6, which correspond to three separate mice in the experiment. A and B demonstrated high- and low-responding, respectively, to acute (Day 1) methamphetamine treatment. (The mean response in animals administered saline was less than 10,000 cm on each day.) Over the remaining days, the drug-induced hyperactivity persisted and the development of sensitization to the hyperactivity was evident by Day 12. However, C displayed heightened locomotor activity on Day 1, followed by little hyperactivity on Days 2 – 4, and a return to heightened levels on Days 5 and 12. These data are consistent with other findings (Bevins & Peterson, 2004) and could be used to model and study the individual differences in response to stimulants observed in humans (Comings & Blum, 2000; Haile et al., 2009). For example, Dietz and colleagues (2005) observed that individual differences in amphetamine sensitization are related to differences in dopamine transporter activity (Dietz et al., 2005).

Table 3. Examples of locomotor sensitization studies in mice

Mouse Strain	Parameters & Dose	Relevant Findings
ICR	Mice were tested each day: Days 1–5, 1 mg/kg methamphetamine; Days 6-10, no treatment; Day 11, saline treatment; Days 12-14, no treatment; Day 15, methamphetamine.	Landa et al (2006) showed that locomotor sensitization develops to methamphetamine, and this effect was attenuated by cannabinoid receptor ligands
C57BL/6J	Mice were tested every-other day: Days 1-14, 1-2 mg/kg methamphetamine; Days 15-21, no treatment; Day 22, methamphetamine.	Fukushima et al (2007) reported that locomotor sensitization develops to methamphetamine, and this effect was altered in knock-out mice.
Kumming	Mice were tested each day: Days 1-7, 2 mg/kg methamphetamine; Days 8-14, no treatment; Day15, methamphetamine	Li et al (2005) reported that sensitization develops to methamphetamine, and its initiation and expression were mediated by GABA receptors.
CD-1	Mice were tested each day: Days 1-7, 2 mg/kg methamphetamine	Kubota et al (2002) showed sensitization to methamphetamine in histidine decarboxylase knock-out and wild-type mice
ICR	Mice were tested each day: Day 1, saline treatment; Days 2-6, 1 mg/kg methamphetamine; Days 7-10, experimental ligand without methamphetamine; Day 11, experimental ligand and methamphetamine	Kitanka et al (2005) showed sensitization to methamphetamine that was prevented with a monoamine oxidase inhibitor.
C57BL/6J	Mice were tested each day: Days 1-7, 0.62 mg/kg methamphetamine; Days 8-14, no treatment; Day 15, methamphetamine	Shen et al (2010) showed sensitization to methamphetamine that did not develop in opiate receptor knock-out mice.

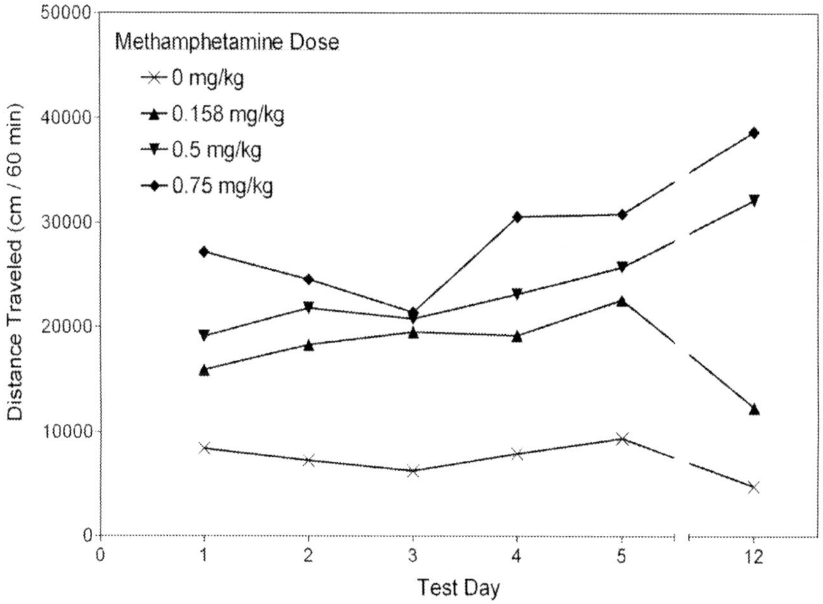

Figure 5. Sensitization develops to methamphetamine-induced hyperactivity in mice. For five consecutive days (Days 1 – 5), male CD-1 mice were placed in an automated activity monitor for 60 minutes and then injected (i.p.) with methamphetamine (0.158, 0.5 or 0.75 mg/kg) or saline (0 mg/kg) and returned to the monitor for 60 minutes. Mice were not tested on the next 6 days (Days 6 – 11) and were reintroduced to the experimental procedures on Day 12. Data represent mean (±S.E.M.) distance traveled summed across the 60-minute post-injection period. These data, presented as distance traveled in 5-minute intervals, are depicted in Figure 4.

Factors for the Design and Conduct of Sensitization Experiments

Studying the "drug-naïve" rodent compared to the "drug-addicted" rodent in the sensitization model, provides flexibility in experimental parameters (e.g. ease and short duration of protocol), precision and control in experimental manipulations (i.e., pharmacological agents and transgenic procedures), and allows the conduct of research that is not possible to carryout in human subjects. Table 3 provides an overview and summary of a variety of parameters that have been used with mice in different reports in the literature. Within the table is a list of mouse strains, experimental parameters, methamphetamine doses, and relevant experimental findings *via* the procedures used.

Biological and Theoretical Basis of Sensitization

An intriguing extension of behavioral sensitization is the concept of cross-sensitization (Ito et al., 2007; Kuczenski & Segal, 2002). Sensitization that develops to Drug A confers a sensitized response to Drug B. For example, Brennan and colleagues (2007) sensitized rats to benzylpiperazine, a stimulant abused for its euphoric properties, or gave rats repeated vehicle treatment. Later, both groups of rats were given methamphetamine, and the benzylpiperazine-treated rats displayed much greater hyperactivity in response to methamphetamine, than the saline-treated rats (Brennan et al., 2007). Typically greater cross-sensitization is observed for drugs of the same pharmacological class (e.g., the stimulants methamphetamine and cocaine), than for drugs across classes (e.g., methamphetamine and the sedative diazepam).

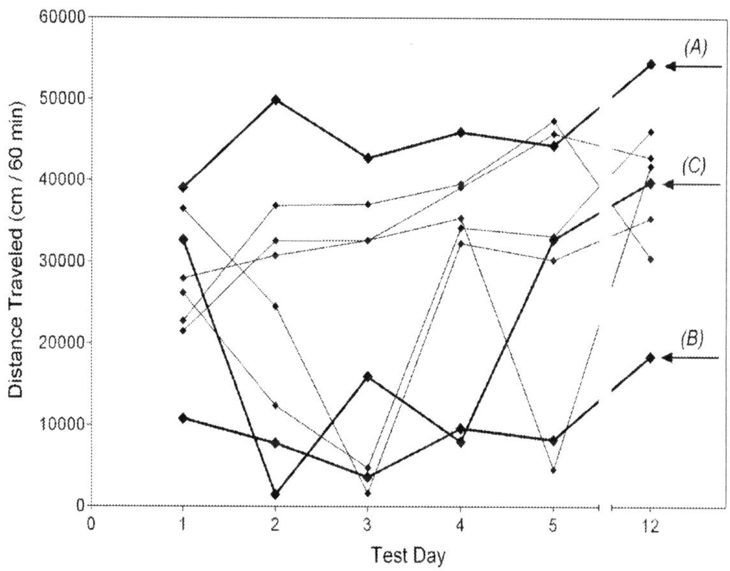

Figure 6. There are individual differences in the development of sensitization to methamphetamine-induced hyperactivity in mice. For five consecutive days (Days 1 – 5), male CD-1 mice were placed in an automated activity monitor for 60 minutes and then injected (i.p.) with methamphetamine (0.5 or 0.75 mg/kg) or saline (0 mg/kg) and returned to the monitor for 60 minutes. Rats were not tested on the next 6 days (Days 6 – 11) and were reintroduced to the experimental procedures on Day 12. Data represent distance traveled summed across the 60-minute post-injection period for each of the mice that received 0.75 mg/kg methamphetamine. A, B and C indicate the activity patterns for three individual mice.

Understanding how abused drugs can cross-sensitize, possibly leaving a user more susceptible to all drugs of abuse, will be very important as research uncovers more information about the shared neural correlates and addictive properties of the vast number of drugs of abuse. Certainly, few if any addicts presently seeking treatment have ever used only one psychoactive substance.

Table 4 provides a summary of studies in the literature that have investigated the mechanisms of action responsible for the initiation and expression of methamphetamine sensitization. Pharmacological and gene knock-out studies (Kitanaka et al., 2005; Fukushima et al., 2007) indicate that dopamine contributes to both the initiation and the expression of methamphetamine sensitization, as would be expected from its theoretical basis (Robinson & Berridge, 1993, 2000, 2001). However, other pharma-cological targets such as cannabinoids (Landa et al., 2006), GABA (Li et al., 2005), histamine (Kubota et al., 2002; Iwabuchi et al., 2004; Okuda et al., 2009), nitric oxide (Itzhak et al., 2000), opioids (Shen et al., 2010), and serotonin (Takamatsu et al., 2006; Ago et al., 2006, 2007, 2008; & Yoo et al., 2010) have also been shown to contribute to methamphetamine sensitization.

Table 4. Signaling systems implicated in methamphetamine sensitization in mice

Signaling System	Mouse Strain	Relevant Findings
Cannabinoid		
	ICR	Landa et al (2006) reported that CB1 (methandamide), but not CB2 (JWH015), cannabinoid receptor agonists result in cross-sensitization to methamphetamine and a CB1 cannabinoid receptor antagonist (AM251) prevented the cross-sensitization.
Dopamine		
	C57BL/6J	Fukushima et al (2007) reported that knock-out of the genes for dopamine storage and release (the dopamine and veiscular transporters), delays the development of sensitization to methamphetamine; however, there is a greater role for the dopamine transporter in methamphetamine sensitization.
	ICR	Kitanka et al (2005) reported that a monoamine oxidase inhibitor (clorgyline) can prevent sensitization to methamphetamine

Signaling System	Mouse Strain	Relevant Findings
GABA		
	Kunning	Li et al (2005) reported a GABA receptor agonist (valproic acid) prevents the initiation and expression of methamphetamine sensitization.
Histamine		
	CD-1	Kubota et al (2002) reported hisitidine decarboxylase knock-out mice enhances methamphetamine sensitization, compared to wild-type mice.
	Not Reported	Iwabuchi et al (2004) reported that methamphetamine-induced sensitization is more pronounced in H1 and H2 histamine receptor knock-out mice, compared to wild-type mice.
	C57BL	Okuda et al (2009) reported no effect of H3 histamine receptors in the development of methamphetamine sensitization
Nitric Oxide		
	C57BL/6J	Itzhak et al (2000) reported that neuronal nitric oxide synthase (NOS) knock-out mice did not display sensitization to methamphetamine, while inducible NOS knock-out mice did display methampehtamine sensitization.
Opioid		
	C57BL	Shen et al (2010) reported μ opiate receptor knock-out mice show decreased initiation and expression of methamphetamine sensitization, compared to wild-type mice.
Serotonin		
	C57BL/6J	Takamatsu et al (2006) reported a serotonin transporter inhibitor (fluoxetine) reduces the initiation of methamphetamine sensitization.
	ddY	Ago et al (2006, 2007, 2008) reported $5\text{-}HT_{1A}$ serotonin receptor agonists (osemezotan) and $5\text{-}HT_2$ serotonin receptor antagonists (ritanserin) diminishes the initation and expression of sensitization to methamphetamine
	ICR	Yoo et al (2010) reported a $5\text{-}HT_3$ serotonin receptor antagonist (MDL 72222) inhibits the initiation of methamphetamine sensitization.

Table 5. Suggested experimental parameters for locomotor activity experiments in mice

Experimental Design		Parameters
Acute Experiments		
	Single Dose	ddY mice receive two habituation sessions (60 min/session). On the test session, a 60-minute habituation session is followed by methamphetamine (2 mg/kg) injection (i.p.) Locomotor activity is monitored for 90 – 120 minutes post-injection in 5 – 10 minute intervals
	Repeated Dose	C57BL mice receive two habituation sessions (60 min/session). On the test session, a 60-minute habituation session is followed by three methamphetamine (5 mg/kg) injections at 2-hour intervals. Locomotor activity is monitored for all/each 120-minute post-injection periods in 10-minute intervals. Observe for neurochemical changes (e.g., change in dopamine metabolism) seven days post-injection.
Sensitization Experiments		
		C57BL mice receive two habituation sessions (60 min/session). On the next seven consecutive days (Days 1 – 7), mice receive methamphetamine (0.75 – 1.5 mg/kg) injection (i.p.) once-daily. Mice are not injected or tested on the following seven days (Days 8 – 14). On Day 15, mice receive methamphetamine to test the expression and/or initiation of sensitization to methamphetamine-induced hyperactivity.

CONCLUSION

Methamphetamine treatment to rodents produces a transient and dose-dependent change in locomotor activity that can be observed, systematically measured and analyzed statistically. With repeated methamphetamine treatment, sensitization develops to the hyperactivity. Both the effects of acute and repeated methamphetamine administration can be altered by agents active in the central nervous system. Several psychological and biological theories provide a basis to use locomotor activity as a tool to study methamphetamine abuse, dependence and addiction.

As with any experimental procedure, each research lab needs to establish the experimental procedures that produce reliable locomotor hyperactivity and/or sensitization to drug-induced hyperactivity. The research hypothesis and variables to be manipulated (e.g., use of gene knock-out mice or pharmacological agents) will also inform the experimental design. For example, if Treatment X is expected to decrease methamphetamine-induced hyperactivity, a more robust methamphetamine-induced hyperactivity should be induced initially to observe the treatment's inhibitory effect. Based on areview of the literature, Table 5 provides suggested experimental parameters (e.g., habituation sessions and methamphetamine doses) for acute and sensitization experiments in mice.

ACKNOWLEDGMENT

The authors' research on psychostimulant addiction is supported partially by a grant from the National Institute on Drug Abuse (DA028477) to John R. Lever, Susan Z. Lever and Dennis K. Miller at the University of Missouri. The authors appreciate the contributions of Clark E. Oelrichs, Ashley N. Simmons, Stephanie L. Myer, and Derick C. Davis to our laboratory's locomotor activity work.

REFERENCES

Ago, Y., Arikawa, S., Yata, M., Yano, K., Abe, M., Takuma, K., et al. (2009). Role of prefrontal dopaminergic neurotransmission in glucocorticoid receptor-mediated modulation of methamphetamine-induced hyperactivity. *Synapse, 63*(1), 7-14.

Ago, Y., Nakamura, S., Baba, A., & Matsuda, T. (2008). Neuropsychotoxicity of abused drugs: effects of serotonin receptor ligands on methamphetamine- and cocaine-induced behavioral sensitization in mice. *J Pharmacol Sci, 106*(1), 15-21.

Ago, Y., Nakamura, S., Kajita, N., Uda, M., Hashimoto, H., Baba, A., et al. (2007). Ritanserin reverses repeated methamphetamine-induced behavioral and neurochemical sensitization in mice. *Synapse, 61*(9), 757-763.

Ago, Y., Nakamura, S., Uda, M., Kajii, Y., Abe, M., Baba, A., et al. (2006). Attenuation by the 5-HT1A receptor agonist osemozotan of the behavioral effects of single and repeated methamphetamine in mice. *Neuropharmacology, 51*(4), 914-922.

Bardo, M. T., Donohew, R. L., & Harrington, N. G. (1996). Psychobiology of novelty seeking and drug seeking behavior. *Behavioral Brain Research, 77*, 23-43.

Bevins, R. A., & Peterson, J. L. (2004). Individual differences in rats' reactivity to novelty and the unconditioned and conditioned locomotor effects of methamphetamine. *Pharmacol Biochem Behav, 79*(1), 65-74.

Brennan, K., Johnstone, A., Fitzmaurice, P., Lea, R., & Schenk, S. (2007). Chronic benzylpiperazine (BZP) exposure produces behavioral sensitization and cross-sensitization to methamphetamine (MA). *Drug Alcohol Depend, 88*(2-3), 204-213.

Byrnes-Blake, K. A., Laurenzana, E. M., Carroll, F. I., Abraham, P., Gentry, W. B., Landes, R. D., et al. (2003). Pharmacodynamic mechanisms of monoclonal antibody-based antagonism of (+)-methamphetamine in rats. *Eur J Pharmacol, 461*(2-3), 119-128.

Camarasa, J., Rates, S. G., Pubill, D., & Escubedo, E. (2009). The involvement of nicotinic receptor subtypes in the locomotor activity and analgesia induced by methamphetamine in mice. *Behav Pharmacol, 20*(7), 623-630.

Comings, D. E., & Blum, K. (2000). Reward deficiency syndrome: genetic aspects of behavioral disorders. *Prog Brain Res, 126*, 325-341.

Dluzen, D. E., & Liu, B. (2008). Gender differences in methamphetamine use and responses: a review. *Gend Med, 5*(1), 24-35.

Dobbs, L. K., & Mark, G. P. (2008). Comparison of systemic and local methamphetamine treatment on acetylcholine and dopamine levels in the ventral tegmental area in the mouse. *Neuroscience, 156*(3), 700-711.

Fornai, F., Biagioni, F., Fulceri, F., Murri, L., Ruggieri, S., & Paparelli, A. (2009). Intermittent Dopaminergic stimulation causes behavioral sensitization in the addicted brain and parkinsonism. *Int Rev Neurobiol, 88*, 371-398.

Fukushima, S., Shen, H., Hata, H., Ohara, A., Ohmi, K., Ikeda, K., et al. (2007). Methamphetamine-induced locomotor activity and sensitization in dopamine transporter and vesicular monoamine transporter 2 double mutant mice. *Psychopharmacology (Berl), 193*(1), 55-62.

Ginawi, O. T., Al-Majed, A. A., & Al-Suwailem, A. K. (2005). NAN-190, a possible specific antagonist for methamphetamine. *Regul Toxicol Pharmacol, 41*(2), 122-127.

Ginawi, O. T., Al-Majed, A. A., Al-Suwailem, A. K., & El-Hadiyah, T. M. (2004). Involvement of some 5-HT receptors in methamphetamine-induced locomotor activity in mice. *J Physiol Pharmacol, 55*(2), 357-369.

Glickstein, S. B., & Schmauss, C. (2004). Effect of methamphetamine on cognition and repetitive motor behavior of mice deficient for dopamine D2 and D3 receptors. *Ann N Y Acad Sci, 1025*, 110-118.

Glickstein, S. B., & Schmauss, C. (2004). Focused motor stereotypies do not require enhanced activation of neurons in striosomes. *J Comp Neurol, 469*(2), 227-238.

Graybiel, A. M., Aosaki, T., Flaherty, A. W., & Kimura, M. (1994). The basal ganglia and adaptive motor control. *Science, 265*(5180), 1826-1831.

Hagino, Y., Kasai, S., Han, W., Yamamoto, H., Nabeshima, T., Mishina, M., et al. (2010). Essential role of NMDA receptor channel epsilon4 subunit (GluN2D) in the effects of phencyclidine, but not methamphetamine. *PLoS One, 5*(10), e13722.

Haile, C. N., Kosten, T. R., & Kosten, T. A. (2009). Pharmacogenetic treatments for drug addiction: cocaine, amphetamine and methamphetamine. *Am J Drug Alcohol Abuse, 35*(3), 161-177.

Hunt, D., (2006). *Methamphetamine Abuse: Challenges for Law Enforcement and Communities* (NCJ 214117). National Institute of Justice (NIJ), Washington, DC: Government Printing Office.

Inoue, I., Yanai, K., Kitamura, D., Taniuchi, I., Kobayashi, T., Niimura, K., et al. (1996). Impaired locomotor activity and exploratory behavior in mice lacking histamine H1 receptors. *Proc Natl Acad Sci U S A, 93*(23), 13316-13320.

Ishiguro, H., Horiuchi, Y., Ishikawa, M., Koga, M., Imai, K., Suzuki, Y., et al. (2010). Brain cannabinoid CB2 receptor in schizophrenia. *Biol Psychiatry, 67*(10), 974-982.

Ito, S., Mori, T., Namiki, M., Suzuki, T., & Sawaguchi, T. (2007). Complicated interaction between psychostimulants and morphine in expression of phenotype of behavior in the dopaminergic system of BALB/c mice. *J Pharmacol Sci, 105*(4), 326-333.

Itzhak, Y., Martin, J. L., & Ali, S. F. (2000). Comparison between the role of the neuronal and inducible nitric oxide synthase in methamphetamine-induced neurotoxicity and sensitization. *Ann N Y Acad Sci, 914*, 104-111.

Iwabuchi, K., Kubota, Y., Ito, C., Watanabe, T., & Yanai, K. (2004). Methamphetamine and brain histamine: a study using histamine-related gene knockout mice. *Ann N Y Acad Sci, 1025*, 129-134.

Kandel, E. R., Schwartz, J. H., & Jessell, T. M. (1995). Essentials of neural science and behavior. McGraw-Hill Professional.

Kamens, H. M., & Phillips, T. J. (2008). A role for neuronal nicotinic acetylcholine receptors in ethanol-induced stimulation, but not cocaine- or methamphetamine-induced stimulation. *Psychopharmacology (Berl), 196*(3), 377-387.

Kelly, M. A., Low, M. J., Rubinstein, M., & Phillips, T. J. (2008). Role of dopamine D1-like receptors in methamphetamine locomotor responses of D2 receptor knockout mice. *Genes Brain Behav, 7*(5), 568-577.

Kitanaka, N., Kitanaka, J., & Takemura, M. (2005). Repeated clorgyline treatment inhibits methamphetamine-induced behavioral sensitization in mice. *Neurochem Res, 30*(4), 445-451.

Kobayashi, K., & Sano, H. (2000). Dopamine deficiency in mice. *Brain Dev, 22 Suppl 1*, S54-60.

Krasnova, I. N., Betts, E. S., Dada, A., Jefferson, A., Ladenheim, B., Becker, K. G., et al. (2007). Neonatal dopamine depletion induces changes in morphogenesis and gene expression in the developing cortex. *Neurotox Res, 11*(2), 107-130.

Krasnova, I. N., Hodges, A. B., Ladenheim, B., Rhoades, R., Phillip, C. G., Cesena, A., et al. (2009). Methamphetamine treatment causes delayed decrease in novelty-induced locomotor activity in mice. *Neurosci Res, 65*(2), 160-165.

Kubota, Y., Ito, C., Sakurai, E., Watanabe, T., & Ohtsu, H. (2002). Increased methamphetamine-induced locomotor activity and behavioral sensitization in histamine-deficient mice. *J Neurochem, 83*(4), 837-845.

Kuczenski, R., & Segal, D. S. (2002). Exposure of adolescent rats to oral methylphenidate: preferential effects on extracellular norepinephrine and absence of sensitization and cross-sensitization to methamphetamine. *J Neurosci, 22*(16), 7264-7271.

Landa, L., Slais, K., & Sulcova, A. (2006). Impact of cannabinoid receptor ligands on behavioural sensitization to antiaggressive methamphetamine effects in the model of mouse agonistic behaviour. *Neuro Endocrinol Lett, 27*(6), 703-710.

Li, J. X., Han, R., Deng, Y. P., Chen, S. Q., & Liang, J. H. (2005). Different effects of valproate on methamphetamine- and cocaine-induced behavioral sensitization in mice. *Behav Brain Res, 161*(1), 125-132.

Matsumoto, R. R., Shaikh, J., Wilson, L. L., Vedam, S., & Coop, A. (2008). Attenuation of methamphetamine-induced effects through the antagonism of sigma (sigma) receptors: Evidence from in vivo and in vitro studies. *Eur Neuropsychopharmacol, 18*(12), 871-881.

Mori, T., Ito, S., Kita, T., Narita, M., Suzuki, T., & Sawaguchi, T. (2006). Effects of mu-, delta- and kappa-opioid receptor agonists on methamphetamine-induced self-injurious behavior in mice. *Eur J Pharmacol, 532*(1-2), 81-87.

Nakagawa, T., Fujio, M., Ozawa, T., Minami, M., & Satoh, M. (2005). Effect of MS-153, a glutamate transporter activator, on the conditioned rewarding effects of morphine, methamphetamine and cocaine in mice. *Behav Brain Res, 156*(2), 233-239.

Nguyen, E. C., McCracken, K. A., Liu, Y., Pouw, B., & Matsumoto, R. R. (2005). Involvement of sigma (sigma) receptors in the acute actions of methamphetamine: receptor binding and behavioral studies. *Neuro-pharmacology, 49*(5), 638-645.

Okuda, T., Zhang, D., Shao, H., Okamura, N., Takino, N., Iwamura, T., et al. (2009). Methamphetamine- and 3,4-methylenedioxymethamphetamine-induced behavioral changes in histamine H3-receptor knockout mice. *J Pharmacol Sci, 111*(2), 167-174.

Okuyama, S., Chaki, S., Yoshikawa, R., Suzuki, Y., Ogawa, S., Imagawa, Y., et al. (1997). In vitro and in vivo characterization of the dopamine D4 receptor, serotonin 5-HT2A receptor and alpha-1 adrenoceptor antagonist (R)-(+)-2-amino-4-(4-fluorophenyl)-5-[1-[4-(4-fluorophenyl)-4-oxobutyl] pyrrolidin-3-yl]thiazole (NRA0045). *J Pharmacol Exp Ther, 282*(1), 56-63.

Picard, M., Morisset, S., Cloix, J. F., Bizot, J. C., Guerin, M., Beneteau, V., et al. (2010). Pharmacological, neurochemical, and behavioral profile of JB-788, a new 5-HT1A agonist. *Neuroscience, 169*(3), 1337-1346.

Pickens, R., & Thompson, T. (1968). Cocaine-reinforced behavior in rats: effects of reinforcement magnitude and fixed-ratio size. *J Pharmacol Exp Ther, 161*(1), 122-129.

Polston, J. E., Cunningham, C. S., Rodvelt, K. R., & Miller, D. K. (2006). Lobeline augments and inhibits cocaine-induced hyperactivity in rats. *Life Sci, 79*(10), 981-990.

Robinson, T. E., & Berridge, K. C. (1993). The neural basis of drug craving: an incentive-sensitization theory of addiction. *Brain Research Reviews, 18*(3), 247-291.

Robinson, T. E., & Berridge, K. C. (2000). The psychology and neurobiology of addiction: an incentive-sensitization view. *Addiction, 95*, S91-S117.

Robinson, T. E., & Berridge, K. C. (2001). Mechanisms of action of addictive stimuli: Incentive-sensitization and addiction. *Addiction, 96*, 103-114.

Rodvelt, K. R., Oelrichs, C. E., Blount, L. R., Fan, K. H., Lever, S. Z., Lever, J. R., et al. (2011). The sigma receptor agonist SA4503 both attenuates and enhances the effects of methamphetamine. *Drug Alcohol Depend.*

Rubinstein, M., Phillips, T. J., Bunzow, J. R., Falzone, T. L., Dziewczapolski, G., Zhang, G., et al. (1997). Mice lacking dopamine D4 receptors are supersensitive to ethanol, cocaine, and methamphetamine. *Cell, 90*(6), 991-1001.

Scibelli, A. C., McKinnon, C. S., Reed, C., Burkhart-Kasch, S., Li, N., Baba, H., et al. (2011). Selective breeding for magnitude of methamphetamine-induced sensitization alters methamphetamine consumption. *Psychopharmacology (Berl), 214*(4), 791-804.

Shadrina, M. I., Slominsky, P. A., & Limborska, S. A. (2010). Molecular mechanisms of pathogenesis of Parkinson's disease. *Int Rev Cell Mol Biol, 281*, 229-266.

Shen, X., Purser, C., Tien, L. T., Chiu, C. T., Paul, I. A., Baker, R., et al. (2010). mu-Opioid receptor knockout mice are insensitive to methamphetamine-induced behavioral sensitization. *J Neurosci Res, 88*(10), 2294-2302.

Shimosato, K., Nagao, N., Watanabe, S., & Kitayama, S. (2003). Suppressive effects of trihexyphenidyl on methamphetamine-induced dopamine release as measured by in vivo microdialysis. *Synapse, 49*(1), 47-54.

Shimosato, K., Watanabe, S., & Kitayama, S. (2001). Differential effects of trihexyphenidyl on place preference conditioning and locomotor stimulant activity of cocaine and methamphetamine. *Naunyn Schmiedebergs Arch Pharmacol, 364*(1), 74-80.

Steinkellner, T., Freissmuth, M., Sitte, H. H., & Montgomery, T. (2011). The ugly side of amphetamines: short- and long-term toxicity of 3,4-methylenedioxymethamphetamine (MDMA, 'Ecstasy'), methamphetamine and D-amphetamine. *Biol Chem, 392*(1-2), 103-115.

Tabibnia, G., Monterosso, J. R., Baicy, K., Aron, A. R., Poldrack, R. A., Chakrapani, S., et al. (2011). Different forms of self-control share a neurocognitive substrate. *J Neurosci, 31*(13), 4805-4810.

Takamatsu, Y., Yamamoto, H., Ogai, Y., Hagino, Y., Markou, A., & Ikeda, K. (2006). Fluoxetine as a potential pharmacotherapy for methamphetamine dependence: studies in mice. *Ann N Y Acad Sci, 1074*, 295-302.

Thomas, D.L. Introduction to Addictive Behaviors (3rd Edition, 2006) New York: The Guilford Press.

Toyota, H., Dugovic, C., Koehl, M., Laposky, A. D., Weber, C., Ngo, K., et al. (2002). Behavioral characterization of mice lacking histamine H(3) receptors. *Mol Pharmacol, 62*(2), 389-397.

Ungard, J. T., Beekman, M., Gasior, M., Carter, R. B., Dijkstra, D., & Witkin, J. M. (2000). Modification of behavioral effects of drugs in mice by neuroactive steroids. *Psychopharmacology (Berl), 148*(4), 336-343.

United Nations Office on Drugs and Crime (U.N.O.D.C.). (2009). *World Drug Report.* United Nations, New York: Government Printing Office.

U.S. Department of Justice (U.S.DoJ), National Drug Intelligence Center. (2010). *National Drug Threat Assessment* (2010-Q0317-001). Johnstown, PA: Government Printing Office.

Vezina, P. (2004). Sensitization of midbrain dopamine neuron reactivity and the self-administration of psychomotor stimulant drugs. *Neurosci Biobehav Rev, 27*(8), 827-839.

Winger, G., Woods, J. H., & Hofmann, F. G. A Handbook on Drug and Alcohol Abuse (4th Edition, 2004) Oxford: Oxford University Press.

Wise, R. A. (1998). Drug-activation of brain reward pathways. *Drug Alcohol Depend, 51*(1-2), 13-22.

Wise, R. A. (2002). Brain reward circuitry: insights from unsensed incentives. *Neuron, 36*(2), 229-240.

Wise, R. A., & Bozarth, M. A. (1987). A psychomotor stimulant theory of addiction. *Psychological Review, 94*(4), 469-492.

Yamanaka, Y., Yamamoto, T., & Egashira, T. (1983). Methamphetamine-induced behavioral effects and releases of brain catecholamines and brain concentrations of methamphetamine in mice. *Jpn J Pharmacol, 33*(1), 33-40.

Yoo, J. H., Lee, H. K., Kim, H. C., Lee, S. Y., & Jang, C. G. (2010). GABA(A) receptors mediate the attenuating effects of a 5-HT(3) receptor antagonist on methamphetamine-induced behavioral sensitization in mice. *Synapse, 64*(4), 274-279.

Yoo, J. H., Nam, Y. S., Lee, S. Y., & Jang, C. G. (2008). Dopamine neurotransmission is involved in the attenuating effects of 5-HT3 receptor antagonist MDL 72222 on acute methamphetamine-induced locomotor hyperactivity in mice. *Synapse, 62*(1), 8-13.

Zombeck, J. A., Gupta, T., & Rhodes, J. S. (2009). Evaluation of a pharmacokinetic hypothesis for reduced locomotor stimulation from methamphetamine and cocaine in adolescent versus adult male C57BL/6J mice. *Psychopharmacology (Berl), 201*(4), 589-599.

Zombeck, J. A., Lewicki, A. D., Patel, K., Gupta, T., & Rhodes, J. S. (2010). Patterns of neural activity associated with differential acute locomotor stimulation to cocaine and methamphetamine in adolescent versus adult male C57BL/6J mice. *Neuroscience, 165*(4), 1087-1099.

In: Methamphetamines
Editors: J. Ornoy and X. He
ISBN: 978-1-62100-244-4

Chapter 3

SIGMA RECEPTORS ARE A POTENTIAL TARGET FOR METHAMPHETAMINE ABUSE AND DEPENDENCE PHARMACOTHERAPIES

Clark E. Oelrichs, Ashley N. Simmons, Stephanie L. Myer, Derick C. Davis, Andrew S. Sage, Kelli R. Rodvelt and Dennis K. Miller*

Department of Psychological Sciences, Center for Translational Neuroscience, and Bond Life Science Center, University of Missouri, Columbia MO, US

ABSTRACT

Sigma receptors have been identified as two subtypes—σ1 and σ2—and are located throughout the brain. The receptors regulate intraneuronal signaling pathways and a number of ligands have been developed to study the receptors' roles in behavior. Several lines of research indicate that σ1 sigma receptor antagonists decrease the behavioral effects of cocaine, and these ligands have been considered potential stimulant addiction pharmacotherapies. An emerging line of research suggests that σ1 and/or σ2 sigma receptors could play a role in the behavioral effects of

* Correspondence: Dennis K. Miller, Department of Psychological Sciences, University of Missouri, McAlester Hall, Columbia MO, 65210, USA. Tel: 573-884-8141, E-mail: millerden@missouri.edu.

methamphetamine. Methamphetamine binds to sigma receptors, and receptor ligands alter the effects of methamphetamine on locomotor behavior in rodents and on dopamine release from neurons. In this chapter, we provide an overview of sigma receptor pharmacology and summarize findings on the interactions between sigma receptor ligands and cocaine, as well as with methamphetamine's *in vitro* and behavioral effects.

INTRODUCTION

Methamphetamine abuse is a significant problem in the United States. It is used by nearly 530,000 Americans ages 12 and older, but the effects are devastating to family and friends of addicts [1]. According to the *Diagnostic and Statistical Manual of Mental Disorders* methamphetamine abuse can cause an array of mental and physical problems when an individual is under its influence such as: anxiety, impaired judgment, anger, vomiting, tachycardia and bradycardia (speeding up and slowing down of the normal heart rate, respectively), seizures, coma and even death [2]. However, methamphetamine withdrawal is just as dangerous, causing fatigue, insomnia and hypersomnia, psychomotor retardation and deep depression that can last several days or weeks. Methamphetamine's withdrawal symptoms make it very difficult for an addicted individual to stop using the drug [3]. Although behavioral therapy is an important component of treatment programs, there is need for a pharmacological agent to reduce physical and psychological withdrawal symptoms and prevent relapse [4]. To develop an effective anti-methamphetamine pharmacotherapy, an understanding of methamphetamine's mechanisms of action and the identification of possible molecular therapeutic targets, are needed.

The underlying neurochemical mechanisms of methamphetamine abuse involve the mesolimbic dopamine system, where methamphetamine causes the release of dopamine from vesicles and presynaptic neurons and activation of pre- and postsynaptic dopamine receptors. (For a review, see the chapter by Davis, Sage and Miller in this volume). While methamphetamine interacts with dopamine transporters and dopamine receptors, it also binds to sigma receptors, indicating that sigma receptors may be involved with methamphetamine's effects in the body.

Sigma Receptors

The sigma receptor was discovered in 1976 by W. R. Martin and colleagues [5] and is now considered a unique protein after first being mistaken as an opioid receptor subtype (e.g., mu, kappa or delta opioid receptors). The sigma receptor has a drug binding selectivity pattern, amino acid sequence, and an anatomical distribution that is distinct from any other known receptor protein [6-8]. Recently, sigma receptors have been considered an important target for pharmacotherapy development, because a remarkably diverse class of ligands—such as antipsychotics, antidepressants, neurosteroids, neuroleptics and psychostimulants (e.g., cocaine and methamphetamine)—bind to sigma receptors with relatively-high affinity [9, 10]. This suggests that sigma receptors could be very important in developing treatments for a range of pathologies, including cocaine and methamphetamine addiction.

There are two sigma receptor subtypes that have been identified and distinguished based on their pharmacological properties—σ1 and σ2 sigma receptors [11, 12]. According to photolabeling studies, σ1 sigma receptors are approximately 25 kDa, while σ2 sigma receptors are smaller at 18-21 kDa [13]. The σ1 sigma receptor was first cloned in 1996 [14] with high homology by using a guinea pig liver, and it has since been cloned [6]. The identification of the amino acid sequences that comprise the σ1 sigma receptor has allowed for a more thorough investigation of ligand-receptor interaction. The σ2 sigma receptor has not been cloned, causing its pharmacological importance to remain less clear.

Both σ1 and σ2 sigma receptors have been identified in peripheral structures such as the heart, kidneys, lungs, testes, ovaries, intestines, muscles and liver [8]. Sigma receptors have also been identified in the central nervous system in many brain structures including the hippocampus, hypothalamus, olfactory bulb and cerebellum [8]. Additionally, both σ1 and σ2 sigma receptors are heavily concentrated in the brain stem, midbrain and limbic system [8]. The limbic region and midbrain are important areas for psychostimulant addiction that include the ventral tegmental area, nucleus accumbens, striatum and substantia nigra [15]. Radioligand binding and immunochemical studies identified σ1 sigma receptors in regions beneath the membrane including the endoplasmic reticulum of neural cells [16]. Compared to other receptor and transporter proteins associated with methamphetamine reinforcement —such as D1 and D2 dopamine receptors and the dopamine transporter—sigma receptors have not been identified in the neuronal membrane at meaningful concentrations.

Sigma Receptor Ligands

The endogenous ligand for sigma receptors has not been identified conclusively; however there are a few prospects, including neuroactive steroids, such as progesterone, dehydroepiandrosterone (DHEA) and pregnenolone [17]. *In vivo* administration of DHEA and pregnenolone inhibited glutamate agonist- N-methyl-D-aspartate (NMDA) stimulated norepinephrine release, suggesting that these steroids function as sigma receptor agonists [18]. In contrast, progesterone inhibited NMDA-stimulated norepinephrine release, and this action was reversed when a σ1 sigma antagonist (BD 1063) was presented, indicating that progesterone works as a σ1 sigma receptor antagonist [19]. Even though these neuroactive steroids work in an "agonist" or "antagonist" fashion on the σ1 sigma receptor, they have relatively-weak affinity (Ki values ≈ 300 nM for pregnenolone and Ki value ≈ 270 nM for progesterone) [19], suggesting that their concentrations in the body may be too low to serve as the primary endogenous sigma receptor ligand.

Another possible endogenous sigma receptor ligand is N,N-dimethyltryptamine (DMT), a naturally-occurring psychedelic found in several plants as well as in the body. It is produced in rat brains when the animal is under stress and is found in human cerebrospinal fluid and blood. DMT is rapidly metabolized so no exact measure of its quantity has been recorded [20]. Similar to the neurosteroids, DMT binds to sigma receptors (Ki values = 24,750 nM for σ1 and 21,700 nM for σ2 sigma receptors), albeit with relatively-low affinity.

Although the endogenous ligand for sigma receptors is not known conclusively, there are many synthetic selective and nonselective sigma receptor ligands. "Selective" ligands have a high affinity for sigma receptors over other receptor types. "Nonselective" ligands may have high affinity for sigma receptors, but share comparable affinity for other receptor types as well. Nonselective ligands may also have affinity for one subtype of sigma receptor over the other (i.e., σ1 versus σ2 subtypes) but may bind to both. Nonselective ligands further complicate matters by producing mixed results when combined with psychostimulants, which complicates the understanding of research on the specific role sigma receptors play in psychostimulant pharmacology.

Table 1. Overview of receptor ligands and their reported affinity for σ1 and σ2 sigma receptors

Ligand	σ1 (Ki value, nM)	σ 2 (Ki value, nM)	σ2 / σ1 Ratio
Agonists			
(+)-3-PPP [21]	79	120	1.5
BD 1031 [22]	1	80	80
DTG [23]	57	22	0.4
PB 28 [24]	0.4	0.7	2
(+)-Pentazocine [25]	2	728	364
PRE 084 [23]	53	32,100	606
SA 4503 [25]	4	63	16
SKF 10,047 [21]	29	33,654	1160
Antagonists			
AC927 [7]	30	138	5
BD 1008 [26]	2	8	4
BD 1047 [26]	1	47	47
BD 1063 [26]	9	449	50
BMY 14802 [27]	265	391	1.5
Haloperidol [28]	3	54	18
LR172 [26]	.4	2	5
MS 377 [29]	73	6,900	94
NE 100 [30]	2	85	43
NPC 16377 [31]	51	55	1.1
Rimacazole [32]	908	302	0.3
SH 3-28 [33]	61	1220	20
Other ligands			
Cocaine [10]	2	31	16
N,N-dimethyltryptamine (DMT) [20]	24,750	21,700	0.9
Methamphetamine [9]	2	47	24

Data in the table reflect Ki values for ligand binding at σ1 and σ2 sigma receptors, as reported in the literature. Typically, affinity for σ1 sigma receptors is determined *via* inhibition of radiolabeled pentazocine binding and affinity for σ2 sigma receptors is determined *via* inhibition of radiolabeled DTG binding.

Table 1 presents an overview of several sigma receptor ligands and their affinity (i.e. Ki value for displacing or inhibiting radioligand binding) for σ1 and σ2 sigma receptors. The ligands' σ2/σ1 sigma receptor binding ratios are also provided as a measure of evaluating selectivity for one subtype over the other. As presented in the table, there are several ligands with greater selectivity for the σ1 over the σ2 sigma receptor subtype (e.g., a σ2/σ1 sigma receptor binding ratio greater than 10), and few with greater selectivity for the σ2 over the σ1 sigma receptor subtype (e.g., a σ2/σ1 sigma receptor binding ratio less than 0.1). The majority of work on the interactions between psychostimulants and sigma receptors has been performed with the selective σ1 sigma receptor ligands. As more selective σ2 sigma receptor ligands are developed and become available commercially, a better understanding of the role that the σ2 sigma subtype plays in cocaine's and methamphetamine's effects will be determined.

Table 1 also identifies the ligands by their action as an agonist or antagonist at sigma receptors. Historically, it has been difficult to classify a ligand conclusively as an agonist or antagonist. Typically, ligands are classified *via* their activity on a protein-coupled receptor (e.g. activating a G-protein) or ion channel (e.g. opening an ion channel). However, sigma receptors are not directly linked to proteins (e.g. D1 dopamine receptors and adenylyl cyclase) or ion channels (e.g., nicotinic acetylcholine receptors and potassium efflux). As such, the "agonist" and "antagonist" labels are inferred by other measures. Sigma receptor antagonists have been classified as those that block the acute effect of cocaine on locomotor activity or convulsions. Agonists usually enhance these effects. The precise pharmacological characterization of sigma ligands as either agonists or antagonists will require the development of a functional assay for these receptors.

Neuronal Mechanisms for Sigma Receptors

The effects of psychostimulants on behavior are related to their abilities to alter neurotransmitter--specifically the monoamines dopamine, norepinephrine and serotonin--storage and release. Sigma receptor ligands have been shown to exert a regulatory role on neurotransmitter release *via* intraneuronal receptors. Monnet and colleagues (1995) investigated neurosteroids that were believed to modulate norepinephrine release through sigma receptor agonism and antagonism [18]. DHEA enhanced NMDA-evoked norepinephrine release, while pregnenolone inhibited it. σ1 Sigma receptor antagonists (BD 1063 and haloperidol) did not alter NMDA-evoked norepinephrine release, but prevented the excitatory and inhibitory effects of DHEA and pregnenolone, respectively. Gonzalez-Alvear and Werling (1994) examined the abilities of sigma ligands to regulate NMDA-evoked dopamine release from striatal slices: Pentazocine and SKF 10,047 inhibited NMDA-evoked dopamine release; however, BD 1008 did not significantly alter NMDA-evoked neurotransmitter release [34]. Overall, these data and other findings (*vide infra*) demonstrate that sigma receptors play a role in drug-induced neurotransmitter storage and release.

The intraneuronal mechanisms for sigma receptors are presented in Figure 1, and it depicts receptor activity during receptor activation *via* low agonist concentrations (left side of Figure) and during receptor depletion (e.g., receptor antagonism or desensitization *via* high agonist concentrations; right side of Figure). Sigma receptors are found in the endoplasmic reticulum of neurons, where they serve as chaperone proteins that assist in the folding and unfolding of other proteins. In the presence of low concentrations of sigma receptor agonists, sigma receptors activate inositol triphosphate (IP3) receptors [8]. This leads to calcium mobilization and generation of adenosine triphosphate—a cellular "energy source" —from mitochondria. IP3 can also be activated *via* activation of neuronal receptors such as the D1 dopamine receptor. Many drugs of abuse, including methamphetamine, indirectly activate D1 dopamine receptors by elevating synaptic dopamine levels [35]. In contrast, when sigma receptors are depleted or blocked by high agonist concentrations, the sigma receptors do not chaperone IP3 receptors [8]. Rather, depletion and blockade contributes to mitochondrial dysfunction and the generation of reactive oxygen species. Inhibition of ion channels in the neuronal membrane might also be observed, which would change the neuron's membrane potential and firing pattern.

Through these processes, sigma receptor ligands could modulate the activity of a variety of receptor proteins associated with drug abuse and dependence, including D1 dopamine receptors and ionotropic glutamate (e.g., NMDA) receptors. Moreover, sigma receptors may regulate the generation of the reactive oxygen species that contribute to methamphetamine-induced neurotoxicity.

SIGMA RECEPTORS AND COCAINE

Like methamphetamine, cocaine is highly addictive and dangerous, and there is a need for pharmacotherapies to block its euphoric effects, minimize dependency, and prevent relapse to drug use following abstinence [36]. Cocaine increases dopamine levels in the brain by inhibiting the dopamine transporter [37]. Importantly, several studies have shown that cocaine interacts with sigma receptors and that sigma receptor agonists and antagonists enhance and inhibit, respectively, cocaine's behavioral and neurochemical effects.

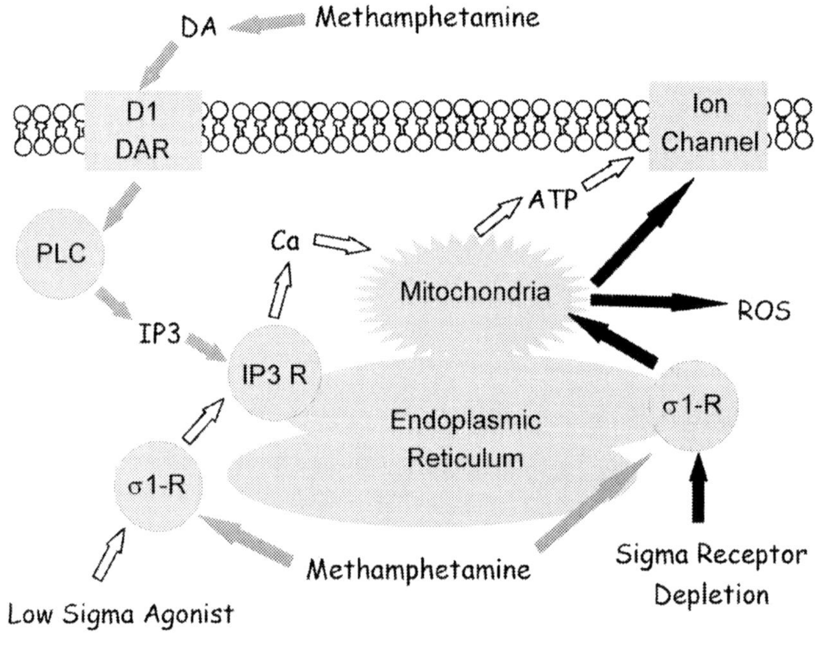

Figure 1. Sigma receptors are located intraneuronally and play a role in signaling. σ1 Sigma receptors (σ1-R) are located in the endoplasmic reticulum of neurons. In the presence of low sigma receptor agonist concentrations (left side), sigma receptors generate calcium (Ca) and adenosine triphosphate (ATP) from inositol triphosphate (IP3). During sigma receptor depletion (right side), neuronal ion channels can be inhibited and neurotoxic reactive oxygen species (ROS) can be generated. Methamphetamine interacts with this mechanism by binding to sigma receptors or by increasing IP3 levels through extra-neuronal dopamine (DA) binding to dopamine receptors (D1 DAR) and activating phospholipase C (PLC).

Cocaine is believed to produce its behavioral effects by binding to (Ki value ≈ 300 nM, [37, 38] and inhibiting the activity of the dopamine transporter; however, cocaine also binds to σ1 (Ki value ≈ 2000 nM) and σ2 (Ki value ≈ 30,000 nM) sigma receptors [10]. There is a ~7-fold difference in binding affinity for cocaine for the dopamine transporter and σ1 sigma receptors and a ~100-fold difference in affinity for the dopamine transporter and σ2 sigma receptors. While cocaine has a greater affinity for the dopamine transporter over sigma receptors, its affinity suggests that cocaine's behavioral effects may be mediated, at least in part, by its interaction with sigma receptors. In addition to the findings from radioligand binding studies, behavioral experiments with sigma receptor ligands and antisense oligodeoxynucleotides also suggest that the effects of cocaine may be mediated by sigma receptors.

With acute and repeated treatment to rodents, cocaine produces a significant transient and dose-dependent increase in locomotor activity [39]. Several studies have shown that pretreatment with σ1 sigma receptor antagonists before cocaine injection attenuates or completely blocks the stimulant-induced increase in locomotor activity. For example, in a recent (unpublished) study in our laboratory, male CD-1 mice were pretreated with the σ1 sigma receptor antagonist BD 1063 (31.6 μmol/kg) 15 minutes prior to a cocaine (60 μmol/kg) injection. BD 1063 produced a ~24% decrease in cocaine-induced hyperactivity, indicating that a blockade of σ1 sigma receptors diminishes this behavioral effect of cocaine. Similar patterns of inhibition have been reported with the receptor antagonists BD 1047 and LR 172 in mice: Hyperactivity induced by cocaine was attenuated by 36% and 97%, respectively, by these antagonists [26]. In a different study, the nonselective sigma receptor antagonists BMY 14802 and rimcazole attenuated cocaine-induced hyperactivity in mice [40]. In these locomotor activity studies [26, 40], the sigma receptor antagonists diminished cocaine's effects at concentrations that did not have an intrinsic effect on locomotor behavior (e.g., producing hyperactivity), suggesting a specific drug-drug interaction between cocaine and the sigma receptor antagonists. A role for sigma receptors to mediate cocaine-induced changes in locomotor behavior is also indicated *via* receptor antisense oligodeoxynucleotides, where the messenger RNA for the σ1 sigma receptor is inactivated. Cocaine-induced hyperactivity was diminished in mice that received the σ1 sigma receptor antisense oligodeoxynucleotide, relative to control mice [41]. Overall, sigma receptor antagonists decrease the hyperactivity induced by acute cocaine treatment.

This behavioral interaction has been used to label sigma receptor ligands as "antagonists".

With repeated cocaine treatment, sensitization can develop to drug-induced hyperactivity. Sensitization is used by animal researchers to model the development of psychological dependence or drug "craving." [35]. Witken and colleagues (1993) reported that the nonselective sigma receptor antagonist NPC 16377 blocked the initiation of cocaine sensitization (i.e., the behavioral transitions that occur during the development of sensitization), but was ineffective against the expression of cocaine sensitization (i.e. the behaviors observed after sensitization has been developed) [42]. However, in another study, the nonselective sigma receptor antagonist BMY 14802 was without effect in altering the development of cocaine sensitization [43].

Cocaine is self-administered by laboratory animals in experiments where the animals are trained in an operant chamber to respond (e.g., press a lever) for drug infusion. This technique is used to study the positive reinforcing properties of drugs [44]. Martin-Farden and colleagues (2007) observed the effects of BD 1047 on cocaine self-administration by male rats: The σ1 sigma receptor antagonist reduced response rates for cocaine infusion, compared to animals that did not receive BD 1047 [45]. In contrast to the effect of the sigma receptor antagonist, sigma receptor agonists potentiate cocaine self-administration, and even maintain self-administration behavior when used as a substitute for cocaine: Hiranita and colleagues (2010) found that both PRE 084 and DTG shifted the cocaine self-administration dose-effect curve to the left, suggesting that both increased the reinforcing effects of cocaine. Moreover, when administered in the absence of cocaine, PRE 084 and DTG yielded response rates that rivaled those observed with cocaine. However, when rats were pretreated with BD 1008 and BD 1047 before PRE 084 or DTG, self-administration rates declined [46]. Overall, these results indicate that sigma receptor agonist, and possibly cocaine, self-administration is mediated by the σ1 sigma receptor.

Conditioned place preference is a technique used to study the role of the contextual cues (e.g., olfactory or visual stimuli) that may be present during drug use and the impact of these cues on subsequent drug-seeking behavior [47]. The sigma receptor has been shown to be a contributing factor in establishing cocaine-induced conditioned place preference. Romieu and colleagues (2002) reported that the σ1 sigma receptor antagonists NE-100 and BD 1047 attenuated the acquisition and expression of cocaine induced conditioned place preference in mice [48]. Neuroactive steroids have affected cocaine-induced conditioned place preference as well: In a 2007 study,

Romieu and colleagues reported that progesterone (sigma receptor antagonist [19]) prevented the development of cocaine- induced conditioned place preference; however, DHEA and pregnenolone (sigma receptor agonists [19]) potentiated this effect when administered before cocaine [49].

Table 2. Summary of the role of sigma receptors in cocaine's effects on behavior

Behavioral Measure	Role of Sigma Receptors
Locomotor activity	Sigma receptor antagonists attenuate cocaine-induced hyperactivity, while sigma receptor agonists augment the locomotor effects of cocaine [26, 40].
Sensitization	Some sigma receptor antagonists (e.g., NPC 16377) block the development of sensitization to the locomotor-activating properties of cocaine [8, 42]
Self-administration	Sigma receptor agonists enhance the positive reinforcing properties of cocaine. Pretreatment with sigma receptor antagonists attenuates the effects of cocaine and decreases the likelihood of cocaine self-administration [13, 45].
Conditioned place preference	Sigma receptor antagonists attenuate the acquisition and expression of conditioned place preference induced by cocaine. Sigma agonists augment the effects of cocaine to develop conditioned place preference [48,49].
Toxicity	Pretreatment with sigma receptor antagonists and antisense oligodeoxynucleotides attenuate convulsions and lethality induced by cocaine. They have also demonstrated the ability to be neuroprotective against cocaine toxicity. Sigma agonists do not create convulsive behavior when administered alone; however, when used as pretreatment with cocaine they enhance and prolong the convulsive behaviors [8, 41].

Cocaine can cause adverse effects such as convulsions, cardiac toxicity and lethality [50]. These effects can be caused by large doses of cocaine or following the development of sensitization to cocaine. σ1 Sigma receptors are found throughout the body, including vital organs, such as the heart, which are adversely affected by cocaine overdose. Over 80% of sigma receptors found in the heart are known to be σ1 sigma receptors [51]. This suggests that convulsive and lethal effects induced by cocaine may be mediated through σ1 sigma receptors. Matsumoto and colleagues (2001) reported that pretreatment with the sigma receptor antagonists BD 1008 and BD 1067 attenuated cocaine-induced convulsions caused by a single, large cocaine dose [52]. Antisense oligodeoxynucleotides also decreased cocaine-induced convulsions [22]. In contrast, pretreatment with the sigma receptor agonists DTG and BD 1031 augmented the severity and increased the duration of cocaine-induced convulsions and stereotypic behaviors associated with drug-induced cardiac toxicity [22].

Several lines of research indicate a pharmacological interaction between sigma receptors and the behavioral effects of cocaine. These findings and general statements on the interactions between sigma receptors and cocaine are presented in Table 2. Generally, σ1 sigma receptor antagonists decrease or inhibit cocaine's effects, while σ1 sigma receptor agonists are found to potentiate cocaine-induced effects and even produce these effects on their own. However, there are still more studies to be conducted on the interactions between cocaine and sigma receptors. Based on the results, sigma receptor ligands could prove to be important pharmacotherapies for cocaine abuse in the future.

Sigma Receptors and Methamphetamine

Methamphetamine creates an intraneuronal pool of dopamine by binding to (Ki value ≈ 100 nM) and blocking the vesicular monoamine transporter (VMAT). The "free" pool of dopamine is then released into the synaptic cleft by methamphetamine binding to (Ki value ≈ 5,000 nM) and reversing the activity of the dopamine transporter [53]. Like cocaine, methamphetamine also binds to σ1 (Ki value ≈ 2,000 nM) and σ2 (Ki value ≈ 47,000 nM) sigma receptors [9]. There is a ~20-fold difference in methamphetamine's binding affinity for the vesicular transporter and σ1 sigma receptors, but methamphetamine binds with equal affinity to the dopamine transporters and σ1 sigma receptors.

Methamphetamine causes an increase in locomotor activity in rodents in a dose-dependent manner. Our laboratory recently determined the effect of the σ1 sigma receptor antagonist BD 1063 on methamphetamine-induced hyperactivity in mice. Male CD-1 mice were acclimated to standard automated activity monitors (Med Associates, St. Albans, VT) for two consecutive days. On the third day, mice were placed in the monitor for 45 minutes, injected (i.p.) with BD-1063 (10 or 31.6 μmol/kg) or saline vehicle, returned to the monitor for 15 minutes, injected (i.p.) with methamphetamine (3.3 or 6.6 μmol/kg) or saline vehicle, and returned to the monitor for 60 minutes.

Figure 2 depicts the distance traveled (in cm) in 5- minute intervals. In the absence of BD 1063, methamphetamine (3.3 and 6.6. μmol/kg) produced a dose-dependent increase in locomotor activity, relative to mice administered only saline (compare solid squares and open squares in the top and bottom panels). Regarding the lower methamphetamine dose (3.3 μmol/kg, top panel), both BD-1063 doses (10 and 31.6 μmol/kg) attenuated methamphetamine-induced hyperactivity. For the higher methamphetamine dose (6.6 μmol/kg), BD 1063 (10 μmol/kg) attenuated the methamphetamine-induced hyperactivity, as well. (The 31.6 μmol/kg BD 1063 dose was not tested against 6.6 μmol/kg methamphetamine). Overall, these data show that antagonism of σ1 sigma receptors diminishes the hyperactivity induced by acute methamphetamine treatment.

Similar findings to those with BD 1063 have been reported in the literature: The receptor antagonists MS-377 and AC 927 as well as sigma receptor antisense oligodeoxynucleotides attenuated methamphetamine-induced hyperactivity in mice [7, 9]. In contrast, σ1 sigma receptor agonists have augmented and inhibited methamphetamine-induced hyperactivity in mice. Rodvelt and colleagues (2011) administered SA 4503 and methamphetamine to rats. Lower SA 4503 doses enhanced methamphetamine-induced hyperactivity, while higher SA 4503 doses attenuated methamphetamine-induced hyperactivity [54]. Generally, these findings suggest that, as observed with cocaine, sigma receptor antagonists diminish the effects of methamphetamine. However, the impact of ligands, that are agonists, on methamphetamine-induced hyperactivity results in a biphasic interaction—enhancement and inhibition of methamphetamine's effects. With repeated drug treatment, sensitization develops to methamphetamine-induced hyperactivity [35]. The sigma receptor antagonists MS-377 and BMY 14802 blocked the development of sensitization to methamphetamine [9, 29]. The sigma receptor agonist (+)-3-PPP augmented methamphetamine-induced hyperactivity in rats sensitized to methamphetamine [55].

The consequences of sigma receptor activation and inhibition on methamphetamine self-administration behavior have not been investigated thoroughly. However, Stefanski and colleagues (2004) reported that methamphetamine self-administration by rats results in an up-regulation of σ1 sigma receptors in the midbrain and limbic regions, relative to rats that were not trained to self-administer methamphetamine [56]. This upregulation is significant because it may cause changes to dopaminergic neurons in the ventral tegmental area--an area where altered neuroplasticity has shown to be important in addictive behaviors [56]. This suggests that σ1 sigma receptors may contribute to the reinforcing properties of methamphetamine, although more self-administration research with receptor ligands is needed. For example, what is the impact of a sigma receptor ligand on the acquisition of methamphetamine self-administration behavior? How do sigma receptors regulate stimulus- (e.g., methamphetamine, stress or contextual cues associated with drug administration) induced reinstatement of drug taking after withdrawal (i.e., the reinstatement model of relapse to drug-taking)? How do sigma receptors affect the incentive value of methamphetamine self-administration (e.g., progressive ratio responding for drug)?

Methamphetamine has neurotoxic effects that can cause damage to monoamine neurons in the brain [35]. Methamphetamine induces oxidative stress, apoptosis and neuronal cell loss. An important contributing factor to the development of neurotoxicity is hyperthermia. Sigma receptor antagonists significantly attenuate methamphetamine-induced hyperthermia. Seminerio and colleagues (2011) reported that the sigma receptor antagonist AC927 attenuated methamphetamine-induced hyperthermia in mice [57]. In contrast, the sigma receptor agonist DTG induced hyperthermia in rats. As such, it is a possibility that the hyperthermia induced by methamphetamine may also be regulated by the sigma receptors, possibly those located in hypothalamus. Sigma receptor ligands have been investigated for their potential role in regulating methamphetamine-induced neurotoxicity, as well. Sigma receptor antagonists inhibited apoptosis and the loss of neuronal terminal buttons following methamphetamine. Matsumoto and colleagues (2008) reported that AC927 attenuated methamphetamine-induced neurotoxicity [7]. In contrast, sigma receptor agonists activated mechanisms that contribute to cell death [58].

Regarding the *in vivo* interaction between sigma receptors and methamphetamine, sigma receptor agonists have been shown to both increase and decrease drug-evoked dopamine release. Liu and colleagues (2001) reported that a series of trishomocubane sigma ligand agonists augmented *d*-amphetamine-evoked dopamine release from rat striatum, which was reversed by sigma receptor antagonists (e.g., BD 1008) [59]. These findings are consistent with a previous study that reported a similar enhancement in *d*-amphetamine-evoked dopamine release by the sigma receptor agonist pentazocine [60]. Our research group recently demonstrated that the sigma receptor agonist SA 4503 inhibits methamphetamine-evoked dopamine release [54].

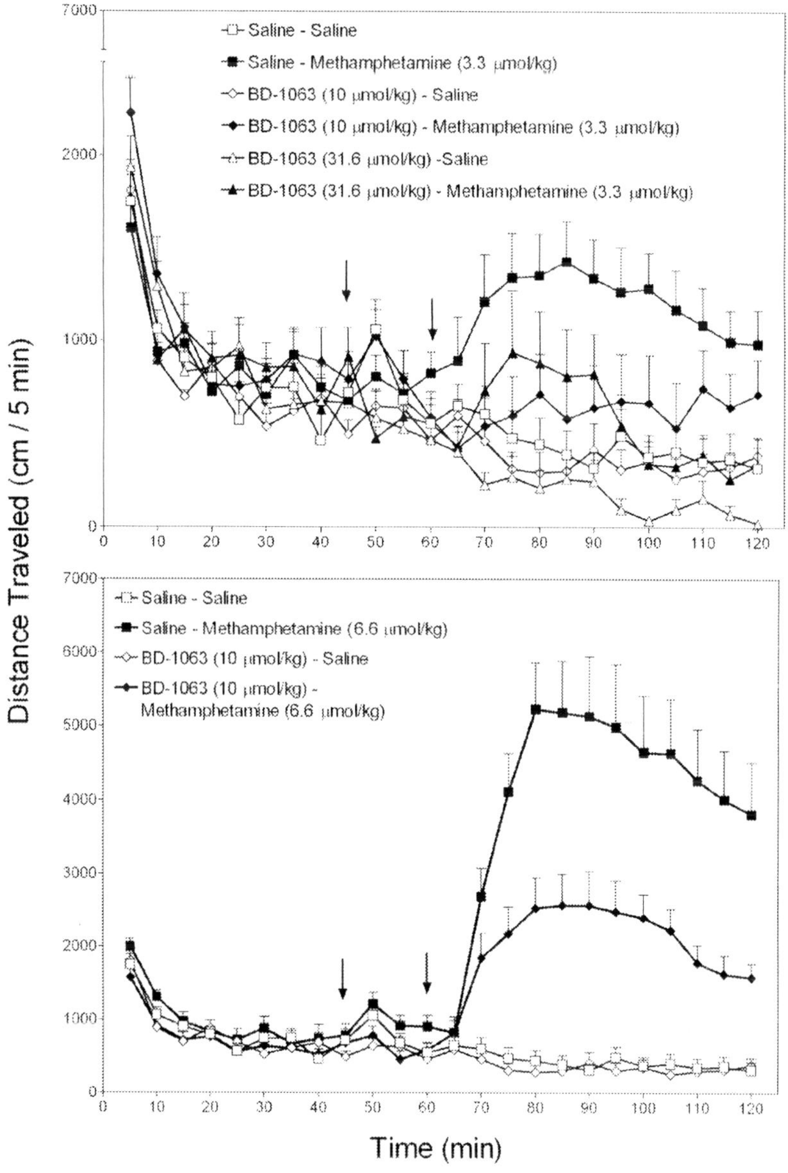

Figure 2. BD 1063 attenuates methamphetamine-induced hyperactivity in mice. Male mice were placed in an automated activity monitor for 45 min, injected (i.p.) with BD 1063 (10 or 31.6 μmol/kg) or saline, returned to the monitor for 15 min, injected (i.p.) with methamphetamine (3.3 or 6.6 μmol/kg) and returned to the monitor for 60 min. Data represent mean (±S.E.M.) distance traveled in 5-min intervals. The left arrow designates BD 1063 injection and the right arrow designates methamphetamine injection. Note the scale of the ordinate differs between the top and bottom panels.

Rat striatal slices were preloaded with [^{3}H]dopamine and superfused in the presence of SA 4503 and methamphetamine (3 or 10 μM). In a concentration-dependent manner, SA 4503 decreased the ability of 3 μM methamphetamine to evoked dopamine release, but did not alter the effect of the higher (10 μM) methamphetamine dose.

Table 3 provides an overview of the role of sigma receptors in methamphetamine's effects on behavior. As observed with cocaine, sigma receptor antagonists diminish the effects of methamphetamine, while receptor agonists enhance methamphetamine's effects.

Table 3. Summary of the role of sigma receptors in methamphetamine's effects on behavior

Behavioral Measure	Role of Sigma Receptors
Locomotor activity	Sigma agonists enhance methamphetamine-induced hyperactivity, while antagonists attenuate these locomotor effects [13, 7, 54, 24].
Sensitization	Sigma receptor antagonists decrease the behavioral sensitization observed after repeated methamphetamine treatment and sigma receptor agonists may enhance sensitization to methamphetamine [29].
Self-administration	Sigma receptors are up-regulated following methamphetamine self-administration [56], which is an opportunity for future testing with sigma 1 antagonists and agonists.
Hyperthermia and neurotoxicity	Sigma receptor antagonists attenuate methamphetamine-induced increases in body temperature, while sigma receptor agonists produce hyperthermia [7]. σ1 sigma receptor antagonists inhibit cell apoptosis caused by methamphetamine, but σ2 sigma receptor agonists may contribute to methamphetamine-induced neurotoxicity. [7, 58]
Neurotransmitter release	Sigma receptor agonists enhance dopamine release in the brain. The impact of receptor agonists and antagonists on stimulant-induced dopamine release remains to be determined [54].

Conclusion

Sigma receptors are found within the central nervous system and are located in areas associated with the reinforcing properties of abused drugs. The development of receptor-selective agonists and antagonists has allowed for investigation of the role of sigma receptors in neural communication and behavior. Generally, sigma receptor antagonists have been shown to diminish the behavioral effects of cocaine and methamphetamine. This suggests a regulatory role for sigma receptors in the development and maintenance of psychostimulant abuse and dependence. As a result, sigma receptor drugs my be developed as pharmacotherapies for drug addiction in the future. However, there is much research that is still needed in animals (e.g., self-administration models of methamphetamine use and relapse) before the findings can translate to humans.

Acknowledgment

The authors' research on psychostimulant addiction is supported partially by a grant from the National Institute on Drug Abuse (DA028477) to John R. Lever, Susan Z. Lever and Dennis K. Miller at the University of Missouri. Derick Davis' participation in research is supported by a grant from the University of Missouri College of Arts and Science Undergraduate Research Mentor Program.

References

[1] Hser, Y. I., Huang, D., Brecht, M.L., Li, L., & Evans, E. (2008). Contrasting trajectories of heroin cocaine, and methamphetamine use. *Journal of Addictive Disorders*, 27(3), 13-21.

[2] American Psychiatric Association. (1994). *Diagnostic and statistical manual of mental disorders* (4th ed.). Washington, DC: Author.

[3] Cho, A. K. & Melega, W. P. (2002). Patterns of methamphetamine use and their consequences. *Journal of Addictive Disorders,* 21(1), 21-34.

[4] Rothman, R. B., Partilla, J. S., Dersch, C. M., Carroll, F. I., Rice, K. C., & Baumann, M. H. (2000). Methamphetamine dependence: medication development efforts based on the dual deficit model of stimulant addiction. *Annals of the New York Academy of Sciences*, 914, 71-81.

[5] Martin, W. R., Eades, C. G., Thompson, J. A., Huppler, R. E., & Gilbert, P. E. (1976) The effects of morphine- and nalorphine- like

drugs in the nondependent and morphine-dependent chronic spinal dog. *Journal of Pharmacology and Experimental Therapeutics,* 197, 517-32.

[6] Brammer, M. K., Gilmore, D. L., & Matsumoto, R. R. (2006). Interactions between 3,4-methylenedioxymethamphetamine and σ_1 receptors. *European Journal of Pharmacology, 553*, 141-145.

[7] Matsumoto, R. R., Shaikh, J., Wilson, L. L., Vedam, S., & Coop, A. (2008). Attenuation of methamphetamine-induced effects through the antagonism of sigma (σ) receptors: Evidence from in vivo and in vitro studies. *European Neuropsychopharmacology,* 18, 871-881

[8] Maurice, T., Martin-Fardon, R., Romieu, P., & Matsumoto, R. R. (2002). Sigma$_1$ (σ_1) receptor antagonists represent a new strategy against cocaine addiction and toxicity. *Neuroscience and Biobehavioral Reviews*, 26, 299-527.

[9] Nguyen, E. C., McCracken, K. A., Liu, Y., Pouw, B., & Matsumoto, R. R. (2005). Involvement of sigma (σ) receptors in the acute actions of methamphetamine: receptor binding and behavioral studies. *Neuropharmacology*, 49, 638-45.

[10] Sharkey, J., Glen, K. A., Wolfe, S., & Kuhar, M. J. (1988). Cocaine binding at σ receptors. *European Journal of Pharmacology,* 149, 171-174.

[11] Lee, I. T., Chen, S., & Schetz, J. A. (2008). An unambiguous assay for the cloned human sigma$_1$ receptor reveals high affinity interactions with dopamine D_4 receptor selective compounds and a distinct structure-affinity relationship for butyrophenones. *European Journal of Pharmacology,* 578, 123-136.

[12] Cormaci, G., Mori, T., Hayashi, T., & Su, T.-P. (2007). Protein kinase A activation down-regulates, whereas extracellular signal-regulated kinase activation up-regulates σ-1 receptors in B-104 cells: Implications for neuroplasticity. *Journal of Pharmacology and Experipemtnal Therapeutics,* 320(1), 202-210.

[13] Cobos, E. J., Entrena, J. M., Nieto, F. R., Cendán, C. M., & Del Pozo, E. (2008). Pharmacology and therapeutic potential of sigma$_1$ receptor ligands. *Current Neuropharmacology*, 6, 344-366.

[14] Maurice, T. & Su, T.-P. (2009). The pharmacology of sigma-1 receptors. *Pharmacology & Therapeutics,* 124, 195-206.

[15] Koob, G. F., Ahmed, S. H., Boutrel, B., Chen, S. A., Kenny, P. J., Markou A., et al. (2004). Neurobiological mechanisms in the transition from drug use to drug dependence. *Neuroscience and Biobehavioral Reviews,* 27(8), 739-749.

[16] Xu, Y.-T., Kaushal, N., Shaikh, J., Wilson, L. L., Mésangeau, C., McCurdy, C. R., et al. (2010). A novel substituted piperazine, CM156, attenuates the stimulant and toxic effects of cocaine in mice. *Journal of Pharmacology and Experimental Therapeutics,* 333(2), 491-500.
[17] Bergeron, R., de Montigny, C., & Debonnel, G. (1999). Pregnancy reduces brain sigma receptor function. *British Journal of Pharmacology,* 127(8), 1769-1778.
[18] Monnet, F. P., Mahe, V., Robel, P., & Baulieu, E. E. (1995). Neurosteroids, via sigma receptors, modulate the [^{3}H]norepinephrine release evoked by N-methyl-D-aspartate in the rat hippocampus. *Proceedings of the National Academy of Sciences* (USA), 92, 3774-8.
[19] Nuwayhid, S. J. & Werling, L. L. (2003). Steroids modulate N-Methyl-D-aspartate-stimulated [^{3}H]dopamine release from rat striatum via σ receptors. *Journal of Pharmacology and Experimental Therapeutics,* 306(3). 934-940.
[20] Fontanilla, D., Johannessen, M., Hajipour, A. R., Cozzi, N. V., Jackson, M. B., & Ruoho, A. E. (2009). The hallucinogen N,N-dimethyltryptamine (DMT) is an endogenous sigma-1 receptor regulator. *Science,* 323, 934-7.
[21] Bowen, W. D., de Costa, B., Hellwell, S. B., Walker, J. M., & Rice, K. C. (1993). [^{3}H]-(+)-Pentazocine: a potent and highly selective benzomorphans-based probe for sigma-1 receptors. *Molecular Neuropharmacology,* 3, 117-126.
[22] Matsumoto, R. R., McCracken, K. A., Pouw, B., Miller, J., Bowden, W. D., Williams, W., et al. (2001). N-alkyl substituted analogs of the s receptor ligand BD1008 and traditional σ receptor ligands affect cocaine-induced convulsions and lethality in mice. *European Journal of Pharmacology,* 411, 261–273.
[23] Garcés-Ramírez, L., Green, J. L., Hiranita, Y., Kopajtic, T. A., Mereu, M., Thomas, A. M., et al. (2011). Sigma receptor agonists: Receptor binding and effects on mesolimbic dopamine neurotransmission assessed by microdialysis. *Biological Psychiatry,* 69, 208-217.
[24] Kitanaka, J., Kitanaka, N., Tatsuta, T., et al. (2009). Sigma 1 receptor antagonists determine the behavioral pattern of the methamphetamine-induced stereotypy in mice. *Psychoparmacology,* 203, 781-92.
[25] Lever, J. R., Gustafson, J. L., Xu, R., Allmon, R. L., & Lever, S. Z. (2006). σ1 and σ2 receptor binding affinity and selectivity of SA4503 and fluoroethyl SA4503. *Synapse,* 59, 350-8.

[26] McCracken, K. A., Bowen, W. A., de Costa, B. R., & Matsumoto, R. R. (1999). Two novel σ receptor ligands, BD1047 and LR172, attenuate cocaine-induced toxicity and locomotor activity. *European Journal of Pharmacology,* 370, 225-232.

[27] Weigl, M., Bedurftig, S., Maier, C. A., & Wunsch, B. (2002). Conformationally constrained ethylenediamines: synthesis and receptor binding of 6,8-diazabicyclo[3.2.2]nonanes. *Bioorganic Medicinal Chemistry,* 10, 2245-57.

[28] Matsumoto, R. R. & Pouw, B. (2000). Correlation between neuroleptic binding to σ1 and σ2 receptors and acute dystonic reactions. European *Journal of Pharmacology,* 401, 155-160.

[29] Takahashi, S., Miwa, T., & Horkiomi, K. (2000). Involvement of σ_1 receptorrs in methamphetamine-induced behavioral sensitization in rats. *Neuroscience Letters,* 289, 21-24.

[30] Chaki, S., Tanaka, M., Muramatsu, M.,& Otomo, S., (1994). NE-100, a novel potent sigma ligand, preferentially binds to sigma 1 binding sites in guinea pig brain. *European Journal of Pharmacology,* 251(1).

[31] Erickson, R. H., Natalie, K. J. Jr., Bock, W., Lu, Z., Farzin, F., Sherrill, R. G., et al. (1992). (Aminoalkoxy)chromones. Selective sigma receptor ligands. *Journal of Medicinal Chemistry,* 35(9), 1526-35.

[32] Husbands, S. M., Izenwasser, S., Kopajtic, T., Bowen, W. D., Vilner, B. J., Katz, J. L., et al. (1999). Structure-activity relationships at the monoamine transporters and σ Receptors for a novel series of 9-[3-(cis-3,5-Dimethyl-1-piperazinyl)-propyl]carbazole (Rimcazole) analogues. *Journal of Medicinal Chemistry,* 42, 4446-4455.

[33] Cao, J., Kulkarni, S. S., Husbands, S. M., Bowen, W. D., Williams, W., Kopajtic, T., et al. (2003). Dual probes for the dopamine transporter and σ_1 receptors: novel Piperazinyl Alkyl-bis(4'-fluorophenyl)amine analogues as potential cocaine-abuse therapeutic agents. *Journal of Medicinal Chemistry,* 46, 2589-2598.

[34] Gonzalez-Alvear, G. M., & Werling, L. L. (1994). Regulation of [^{3}H]dopamine release from rat striatal slices by sigma receptor ligands. *Journal of Pharmacology and Experimental Therapeutics,* 271, 212-219.

[35] Robinson, T. E. & Berridge, K. C. (1993). The neural basis of drug craving: an incentive-sensitization theory of addiction. *Brain Research: Brain Research Reviews,* 18(3), 247-291.

[36] Montoya, I. D. & Vocci, F. (2008). Novel medications to treat addictive disorders. *Current Psychiatry Reports,* 10(5), 392-398.

[37] Schmitt, K. C. & Reith, M. E. (2010). Regulation of the dopamine transporter: aspects relevant to psychostimulant drugs of abuse. *Annals of the New York Academy of Sciences*, 1187, 316-340.

[38] Carroll, F. I., Lewin, A. H., & Mascarella, S. W. (2002). Dopamine-transporter uptake blockers: structure-activity relationships. In Reith M.E.A.(Ed), *Neurotransmitter Transporters*. Totowa, NJ: Humana Press.

[39] Wise, R. A. & Bozarth, M. A. (1987). A psychomotor stimulant theory of addiction. *Psychological Reviews*, 94(4), 469-492.

[40] Menkel, M., Terry, P., Pontecorvo, M., Katz, J. L., & Witkin, J. M. (1991). Selective σ ligands block stimulant effects of cocaine. *European Journal of Pharmacology*, 201, 251-252.

[41] Matsumoto, R. R. & McCracken, K. A. (1999). Antisense oligodexy-nucleotides against σ1 receptors reduce the convulsive and locomotor stimulatory effects of cocaine in mice. *Society for Neuroscience Abstracts*, 25, 303.

[42] Witkin, J. M., Terry, P., Menkel, M., Hickey, P., Pontecorvo, M., Ferkany, J., et al. (1993). Effects of the selective sigma receptor ligand, 6-[6-(4-Hydroxypiperidinyl)hexyloxy]-3-Methylflavone (NPC 16377), on behavioral and toxic effects of cocaine. *Journal of Pharmacology and Experimental Therapeutics*, 266(2), 473-482.

[43] Ujike, H., Kuroda, S., & Otsuki, S. (1996). σ Receptor antagonists block the development of sensitization to cocaine. *European Journal of Pharmacology*, 296, 123-128.

[44] Roberts, D. C., Morgan, D., & Liu, Y. (2007). How to make a rat addicted to cocaine. *Progress in Neuropsychopharmacology and Biological Psychiatry*, 31(8), 1614-1624.

[45] Martin-Fardon, R., Maurice, T., Aujla, H., Bowen, W. D., & Weiss, F. (2007). Differential effects of sigma1 receptor blockade on self administration and conditioned reinstatement motivated by cocaine *vs* natural reward. *Neuropsychopharmacology*, 32, 1967-73.

[46] Hiranita, T., Soto, P. T., Tanda, G., & Katz, J. L. (2010). Reinforcing effects of σ-receptor agonists in rats trained to self-administer cocaine. *Journal of Pharmacology and Experimental Therapeutics*, 332(2), 515-524.

[47] Bardo, M. T., Rowlett, J. K., & Harris, M. J. (1995). Conditioned place preference using opiate and stimulant drugs: a meta-analysis. *Neuroscience and Biobehavioral Reviews*, 19(1), 39-51.

[48] Romieu, P., Phan, V.-L., Martin-Fardon, R., & Maurice, T. (2002). Involvement of the sigma$_1$ receptor in cocaine-induced conditioned place preference: Possible dependence on dopamine uptake blockade. *Neuropsychpharmacology*, 26(4), 444-455.

[49] Romieu, P., Martin-Fardon, R., Bowen, W. D., & Maurice, T. (2003). σ_1 Receptor-related neuroactive steroids modulate cocaine-induced reward. *Journal of Neuroscience,* 23(9), 3572-3576.

[50] Gradman, A. H. (1990). Cardiac effects of cocaine: a review. Yale *Journal of Biological Medicine, 61*(2), 137-147.

[51] O'Brien, C. P., Childress, A. R., Ehrman, R., & Robbins, S. J. (1998).Conditioning factors in drug abuse: can they explain compulsion? *Journal of Psychopharmacology,* 12, 15-22.

[52] Matsumoto, R. R., Gilmore, D. L., Pouw, B., Bowen, W. D., Williams W., Kauser, A., et al. (2004). Novel analogs of the σ receptor ligand BD 1008 attenuate cocaine-induced toxicity in mice. *European Journal of Pharmacology,* 492, 21-26.

[53] Sulzer, D., Sonders, M. S., Poulsen, N. W., & Galli, A. (2005). Mechanism of neurotransmitter release by amphetamines: a review. *Prog Neurobiol,* 75(6), 406-433.

[54] Rodvelt, K. R., Oelrichs, C. E., Blount, L. R., Fan, K.-H., Lever, S. Z., Lever, J. R. et al. (2011). The sigma receptor agonist SA4503 both attenuates and enhances the effects of methamphetamine. *Drug and Alcohol Dependence,* 116(1-3), 203-210

[55] Ujike, H., Tsuchida, K., Akiyama, K., & Otsuki, S. (1992). upersensitivity of σ receptors after repeated administration of cocaine. *Life Sciences,* 51, 31-36.

[56] Stefanski, R., Justinova, Z., Hayashi, T., Takebayashi, M., Goldberg. S. R., & Su, T.P. (2004). Sigma1 receptor upregulation after chronic methamphetamine self-administration in rats: a study with yoked controls. *Pharmacology,* 175, 68-75.

[57] Seminerio, M. J., Kaushal, N., Shaikh, J., Huber, J. D., Coop, A., & Matsumoto, R. R. (2011). Sigma (σ) receptor ligand, AC927 (N-phenethylpiperidine oxalate), attenuates methamphetamine-induced hyperthermia and serotonin damage in mice. *Pharmacology, Biochemistry and Behavior, 98, 12-20.*

[58] Crawford, K. W. & Bowen, W. D. (2002). Sigma-2 receptor agonists activate a novel apoptotic pathway and potentiate antineoplastic drugs in breast tumor cell lines. *Cancer Research,* 62, 313–322.

[59] Liu, X., Nuwayhid, S., Christie, M. J, Kassiou, M., & Werling, L. L. (2001). Trishomocubanes: novel sigma-receptor ligands modulate amphetamine-stimulated [^{3}H]dopamine release. *European Journal of Pharmacology,* 422(1-3), 29-45.

[60] Izenwasser, S., Thompson-Montgomery, D., Deben, S. E., Chowdhury, I. N., & Werling, L. L. (1998). Modulation of amphetamine-stimulated (transporter mediated) dopamine release in vitro by sigma2 receptor agonists and antagonists. *European Journal of Pharmacology*, 346(2-3), 189-196.

In: Methamphetamines
Editors: J. Ornoy and X. He
ISBN: 978-1-62100-244-4

Chapter 4

Methods for Confirmatory Analysis of Methamphetamine in Biological Samples

Stacy D. Brown
Bill Gatton College of Pharmacy at East Tennessee State University, Department of Pharmaceutical Sciences, Johnson City, TN, US

Abstract

Methamphetamine is the most common amphetamine used and, along with 3,4-methylenedioxymethamphetamine (MDMA, Ecstasy), is considered part of a worldwide drug epidemic. Monitoring methamphetamine levels in the body is important for purposes of drug screening for employment, criminal investigations, and therapeutic drug monitoring. While methamphetamine is suitable for detection using immunoassay techniques, these methods tend to have significant cross reactivity with other compounds. Over the last decade, more than eighty different quantitative, confirmatory analytical methods for measuring methamphetamine in biological samples have been published in the scientific literature. Analytical instrumentation used in these methods includes gas chromatography – mass spectrometry (GC-MS), liquid chromatography – mass spectrometry (LC-MS), capillary electrophoresis (CE), among others. These assays are capable of quantifying methamphetamine concentrations in a variety of biological matrices, including blood, plasma, urine, hair, and fingernails. Some of these techniques can achieve detection as low as 0.1 ng/mL (1 ppb) concentrations. The strengths and limitations of these methodologies will be discussed in the context of methamphetamine analysis. Additionally, methods that can simultaneously measure methamphetamine levels as well as metabolites and other drugs of abuse will be highlighted.

INTRODUCTION

Methamphetamine (MAMP) is a small, basic drug molecule amenable to a variety of analytical methodologies (Figure 1). The molecule has one stereogenic center, resulting in enantiomers of different pharmacologic potencies. The D-(+)-methamphetamine has higher abuse potential compared to the L-(-) enantiomer due to its stronger CNS stimulatory activity [1]. Because of this, many published MAMP methods incorporate chiral selectivity as well as sensitivity.

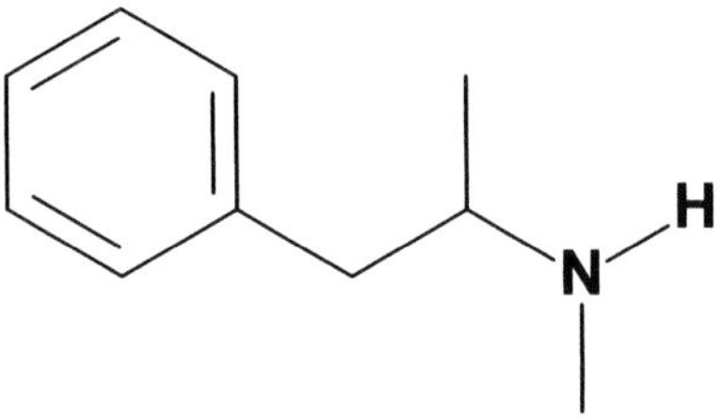

Figure 1. Structure of methamphetamine.

Among the amphetamines, MAMP experiences the highest level of use, likely due to the fact that it is inexpensive and easily manufactured from common ingredients [2]. The demand for sensitive and specific analytical technology for the determination and quantification of MAMP from biological matrices comes from the worlds of forensics, law enforcement, and therapeutic drug monitoring. Because there are legitimate uses for these drugs in treatment of diseases such as ADD/ADHD and narcolepsy, several methods are geared towards pharmacokinetic studies [3-6]. Also, there has been an increase in MAMP drug manufacturing in the US, thus leading to more research dollars spent on monitoring clandestine manufacturing and other criminal activity associated with this drug [7]. Newly published methods for MAMP analysis have averaged 7.5 per year during the last decade, with above average numbers coming out in 2007-2009. Increased interest in this drug has prevailed at the end of the decade due to the emergence of clandestine laboratories for manufacturing MAMP in every state [7].

Sample Matrices and Preparation

Analysis of MAMP is mostly conducted from urine (37% of total methods) and blood related matrices, including whole blood, plasma, and serum (28% of total methods). Many cite the preference of urine over blood due to the non-invasive nature of its collection, and the prevalence of MAMP and metabolites in the urine [8,9]. Along the lines of non-invasive sampling, hair analysis was popular for measuring MAMP concentrations, where it represented 20% of the matrices studied. Some cite the shortcoming of hair analysis to include difficult sample preparation, possible racial bias, and limited available data to correlate to plasma concentrations, yet despite this, hair remains a common matrix for forensic analysis [10]. Saliva analysis was attempted in four MAMP methods [6, 11-13]. In addition, there is evidence to suggest that saliva sampling is well reflective of plasma concentrations of some drugs, including amphetamines. Saliva sampling also shows evidence of drug use quickly after administration [14-16]. Methamphetamine analysis has also attracted the desire to examine some unique matrices including sweat, vitreous humor, meconium, placenta, fingernails, bile, and bone. Some of these unique matrices involve monitoring a mother's drug use during pregnancy [17,18], while others focus on drug concentrations at the site of action [19]. Analysis of human sweat has applications in drug monitoring for rehabilitative purposes, as well as court-ordered and workplace-related drug-free compliance. While the correlation between plasma and sweat concentration of drugs is not well understood, the sweat-based methods tend to be sensitive and able to quantify low ng/patch levels [3,4]. Figure 2 presents a summary of the prevalence of different matrices in the field of methamphetamine analysis.

Liquid-liquid extraction (LLE) separates drugs of interest from the matrix through a partitioning mechanism based on differing solubility in two solvents. Since biological matrices are aqueous based, a less polar organic solvent would be utilized in LLE to drive the analyte molecule out of the biological matrix. Even though LLE is vulnerable to such inconveniences as emulsion formation and poor partitioning of the analyte out of the aqueous phase, it is inexpensive, easy, and dominates the sample preparation arena for methamphetamine methods (36% of all methods). LLE samples are highly suited for gas chromatography separation because the extraction solvents are typically volatile enough for direct injection into the GC without further evaporation or reconstitution. As will be discussed later, GC based methods (including GC-MS) dominate MAMP analysis, thus explaining the high prevalence of LLE to prepare the samples. Most of these LLE preparations intended for GC and GC-MS analysis also involve derivatization. The need for derivatization to enhance volatility suitability for GC separation has led some to advocate the movement of forensic analysis to favor liquid chromatography (LC) over GC [20,21].

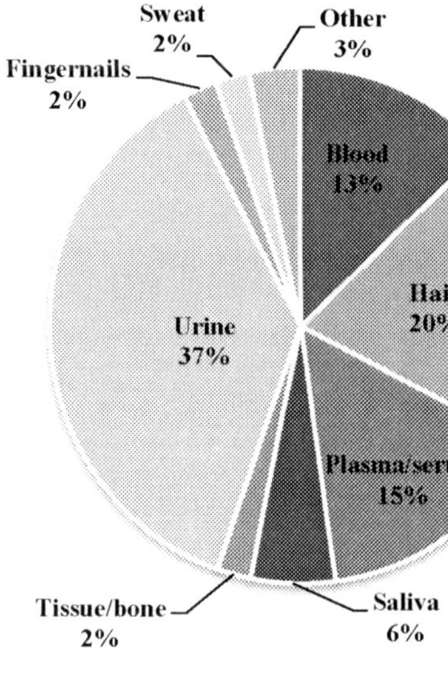

Figure 2. Matrices investigated for methamphetamine analysis.

Solid-phase extraction (SPE) preparations are part of 33% of the MAMP assays from tha last decade. SPE works on a mechanism of partitioning between a solid matrix in a cartridge and a liquid that passes through the solid bed, essentially a scaled-down version of liquid chromatography. Unwanted matrix components are intended to pass through the cartridge bed or be irreversibly retained while the analyte can be selectively eluted and the sample can be subsequently evaporated to dryness and reconstituted in an appropriate solvent and volume for analysis. SPE is more easily automatable, requires lower sample volumes compared to LLE, is more specific than LLE, and typically generates cleaner extracts. While SPE is normally associated with HPLC or LC-MS sample preparation, some of the SPE methods for MAMP prepare samples for GC based analysis, thus also requiring derivatization. A unique SPE approach, called disk SPE, provides an opportunity to reduce solvent consumption while employing a more expeditious extraction of several amphetamine-type substances (ATS) [22]. Some labs used protein precipitation (PP) alone to prepare samples for MAMP analysis [5, 23-25], while others opted for no sample preparation beyond sample dilution [26, 27]. These less scrutinizing ways to prepare samples are better suited to LC-MS methods where no derivatization is required or to capillary electrophoresis (CE) methods. Protein precipitation involves the addition of organic solvent or acid to denature and precipitate proteins. While is can be performed as the sole preparation technique, it commonly precedes an SPE work-up.

Finally, solid-phase microextraction (SPME) is making a substantial mark on sample preparation landscape for MAMP analysis. Solid-phase microextraction (SPME) involves the use of a fiber coated with GC packing material for the extraction of sample molecules from their matrix [28]. The sample molecules are adsorbed onto the fiber and subsequently desorbed into the GC injection port for analysis. The use of SPME as a sample preparation technique was once thought to be limited to volatile analytes. However, advances in sample derivatization with SPME have helped expand the application to non-volatile analytes [29]. SPME is known to be an 'environmentally friendly' sample preparation technique due to its low solvent consumption; however, it also serves as a simultaneous extraction and concentration step. Sixteen percent of the MAMP methods utilize SPME.

Gas Chromatography and Gas Chromatography – Mass Spectrometry

Gas chromatography separations comprised over half (59%) of the total MAMP methods published in the last decade, and of these, 86% utilize mass spectrometric (MS) detection. Gas chromatography separates analytes based on differences in boiling point, which often correlates with molecular weight. Authors cite sensitivity and selectivity as well as compatibility with certain sample preparation techniques (SPME) as reasons for choosing GC [9,30]. Even though GC is more readily available in forensic labs, many authors cite the need for derivatization in GC to be a major drawback [31-35]. While derivatization is not always a prerequisite for GC use, it is required in the case of semi-volatile drugs such as MAMP. Fernandez *et al.* also reports that GC derivatizations are not suitable for some thermally labile compounds [36]. Nevertheless, GC separations remain prominent in MAMP analysis due to the reputation of GC as the 'gold standard' of forensic analysis as well as its high resolution and abundance of literature references.

It comes as no surprise that mass spectrometric detection is dominant in MAMP analysis, both with GC and LC separations. The unique 'fingerprint' data that comprises a mass spectrum enhances its suitability as a confirmatory test for various drugs of abuse. An example mass spectrum of MAMP, acquired following derivatization using pyridine and hexylchloroformate, is shown below in Figure 3. While MAMP and other amphetamines can be easily detected by immunoassay techniques, as a class, they have some of the highest rates of cross reactivity in these types of screening assays [10]. As mass spectrometers have become more easily accessible, as well as easier to use over the last couple of decades, more forensic labs have the finances and expertise to utilize this sensitive and selective technique. Mass spectrometric detection also allows for use of deuterium labeled internal standards for quantification, which removes the possibility of interference with non-analyte related internal standards appearing in a real sample [9,37-39]. Furthermore, mass spectrometric detection provides confirmatory identification as well as quantitative information. Authors cite the complexity of UV chromatograms as a distinct advantage of MS detection [40]. In terms of MS source, one research group provides evidence that atmospheric pressure chemical ionization (APCI) is superior to electrospray ionization (ESI), especially for 3,4-methylene-dioxyamphetamine (MDA), a metabolite used to confirm the presence of MAMP and MDMA [41,42]. Many MAMP methods utilize tandem mass spectrometry or MS/MS techniques to increase sensitivity and selectivity when analyzing complex biological matrices. Even without the application of MS/MS, the use of mass spectrometric detection tends to increase overall sensitivity of a method. For example, the GC methods for MAMP that utilize flame ionization detection (FID) have limits of quantification two-plus orders of magnitude higher than the most sensitive GC-MS methods [43-45]. Conversely, one drawback of mass spectrometric detection involves a suppression of the signal due to interfering ions in the matrix. However, many researchers complete an experiment to demonstrate the absence of ion suppression within their methods [46,47]. An example of one such experiment is shown in Figure 4 below.

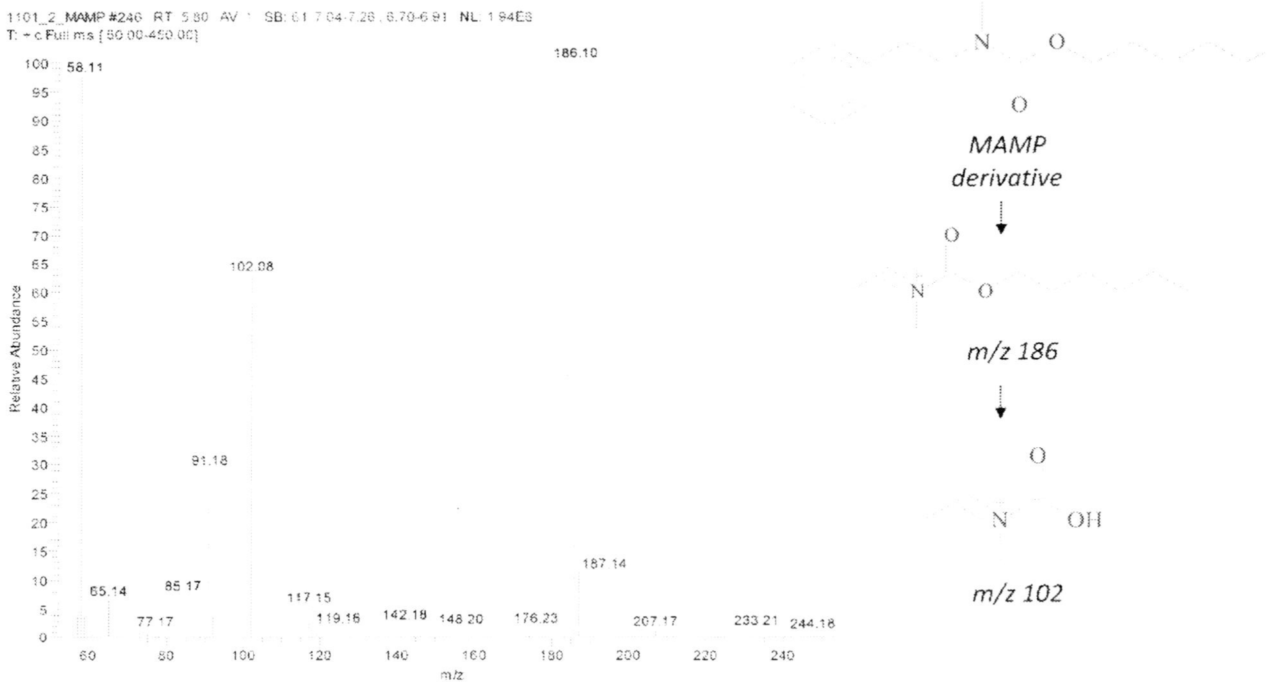

Source: Brown SD, Rhodes DJ, Pritchard BJ. A validated SPME-GC-MS method for simultaneousquantification of club drugs in human urine. Forensic Science International. 2007;171,142-50.[9].

Figure 3. Mass spectrum of MAMP showing the transitions monitored from the extracted ion chromatograms (m/z102,186).

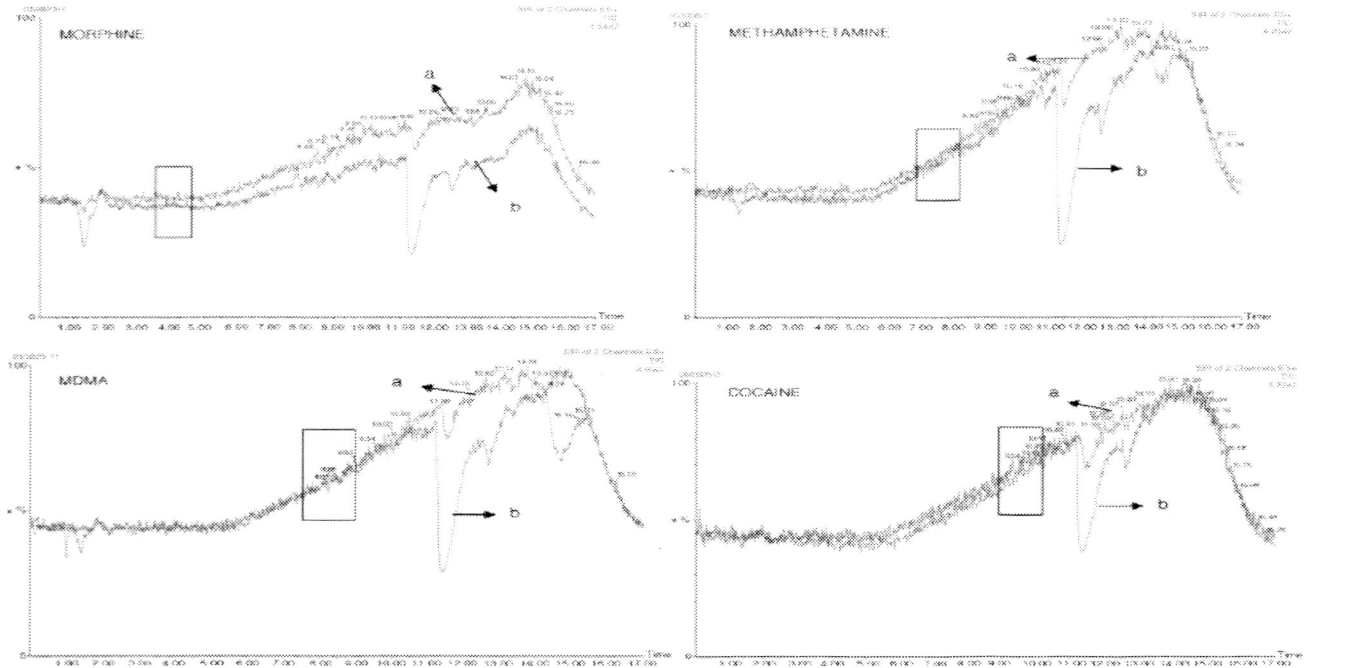

Source: Concheiro M, de Castro A, Quintela O, Lopez-Rivadulla M, Cruz A. Determination of drugs of abuse and their metabolites in human plasma by liquid chromatography-mass spectrometry: An application to 156 road fatalities. *Journal of Chromatography B-Analytical Technologies in the Biomedical and Life Sciences*. 2006;832,81-9. [37]

Figure 4. Evaluation of the ion suppression effect on analyte response by post-column infusion following a mobile phase injection (a) and an extracted blank sample (b). The dotted areas indicate the retention time for the corresponding compound.

Researchers successfully use several different types of derivatization agents to facilitate MAMP's compatibility with GC separation. The most common non-chiral agents include heptafluorobutyric acid anhydride [13,30,34,43,48,49], trifluoroacetic acid anhydride [50,51], and N-methyl-bis(trifluoroacetamide) [52-54]. These derivatizations are coupled with another type of extraction, most commonly LLE, SPE, or SPME. While other agents are mentioned in the literature, one of the most successful chiral derivatizing agents, based on sensitivity achieved, appears to be (2S,4R-N-heptafluorobutyryl-4-heptafluorobutoyloxy-propyl) chloride [55]. This chemical was used to aid in the low pg/mg level quantification of MAMP enantiomers, as well as other amphetamines, in hair (see Figure 5).

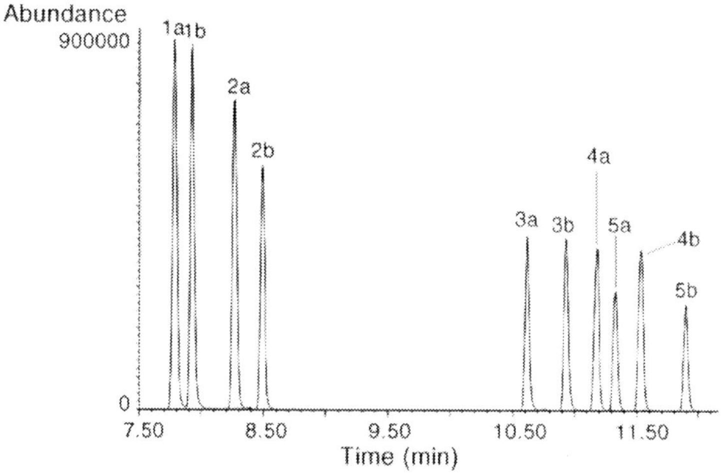

Source: Martins LF, Yegles M, Chung H, Wennig R. Sensitive, rapid and validated gas chromatography/negative ion chemical ionization-mass spectrometry assay including derivatization with a novel chiral agent for the enantioselective quantification of amphetamine type stimulants in hair. *Journal of Chromatography B-Analytical Technologies in the Biomedical and Life Sciences.* 2006;842,98-105. [55]

Figure 5. Selected ion monitoring (SIM) chromatogram of an extract of blank hair spiked with 10 ng/mg of amptehamine type substances (ATS). (1a) (*R*)-amphetamine, m/z 600; (1b) (*S*)-amphetamine; (2a) (*R*)-methamphetamine, m/z 634; (2b) (*S*)-methamphetamine; (3a) (*R*)-3,4-methylenedioxyamphetamine, m/z 664; (3b) (*S*)-3,4-methylenedioxyamphetamine; (4a) (*R*)-3,4-methylenedioxymethamphetamine, m/z 678; (4b) (*S*)-3,4-methylenedioxymethamphetamine; (5a) (*R*)-3,4-methylenedioxy-N-ethylamphetamine, m/z 692; (5b) (*R*)-3,4-methylenedioxy-N-ethylamphetamine.

Liquid Chromatography and Liquid Chromatography – Mass Spectrometry

Liquid chromatographic separations, including those coupled with mass spectrometry and those deemed as ultra-performance liquid chromatography (UPLC) methods, accounted for 32% of separations performed for MAMP assays. Because MAMP is fairly hydrophobic, it is a good candidate for reversed-phase (RP) HPLC separations which rely on a non-polar stationary phase and a moderately polar mobile phase. The separation occurs via a partitioning between adsorption to the hydrophobic column and solubility in the hydrophilic mobile phase. Common stationary phases for this application include silica treated with $(C_8H_{17})(CH_3)_2SiCl$ or $(C_{18}H_{37})(CH_3)_2SiCl$, thus resulting in retention times which are directly related to a compound's polarity, with more non-polar compounds being retained longer.

While mass spectrometry remains the detector of choice to couple with LC separation for MAMP analysis (69% of LC methods), other detection techniques include UV and diode array detection (DAD). These methods rely on an analyte absorbing photons of light within the UV range proportional to the concentration of the analyte. These detection mechanisms are coupled to HPLC, but can also be used for CE systems. They have a selectivity disadvantage when compared to mass spectrometry due to UV absorbance by analytes of interest, as well as the endogenous components of biological matrices. In addition to UV detection or DAD as alternatives to MS as a detector for LC, a few labs utilize derivatization techniques to make MAMP suitable for fluorescence detection [56-60]. When MS is not an available detection technique, FD can provide selectivity over UV but does not always provide a sensitivity advantage. The selectivity of mass spectrometric detection is demonstrated in Figure 6, where the MAMP is not chromatographically resolved from all other amphetamines and drugs of abuse in the assay, yet it can be individually quantified.

Capillary Electrophoresis

Capillary electrophoresis separation was used in 4% of the MAMP methods over the last decade. Electrophoretic separations occur based on the migrations of an ion under the influence of an electric field toward a cathode or anode. CE methods are suitable for ionizable species and are known for high resolution, small sample volumes, and simple method development. Typically, detection occurs by UV absorbance, but due to the low flow rates, CE has also been coupled to MS detection. However, the drawback of interfacing CE with MS lies in the use of buffers to aid in the ionization of analytes for CE separations. For the determination of MAMP, MDMA, and other ATS, Li *et al.* considered the advantage of CE separation [61]. For these authors, CE provides opportunity for a broad range of compound separation while removing the need for compatibility with a stationary phase. To couple the executed method with MS detection, which normally would be incompatible due to the high buffer concentration needed with CE, the authors utilized non-aqueous capillary electrophoresis (NACE). The method was successful in achieving a LOQ of 50 ng/mL from plasma [61]. Jen *et al.* cites the high number of theoretical plates and low sample consumption as an advantage of CE separation [62]. In Figure 7 below, a demonstration of the utility of CE separations is shown for the determination of MAMP and other drugs of abuse in urine. As with chromatographic separations, CE can also supply enantiomeric resolution with the use of β-cyclodextrin in the run buffer [63].

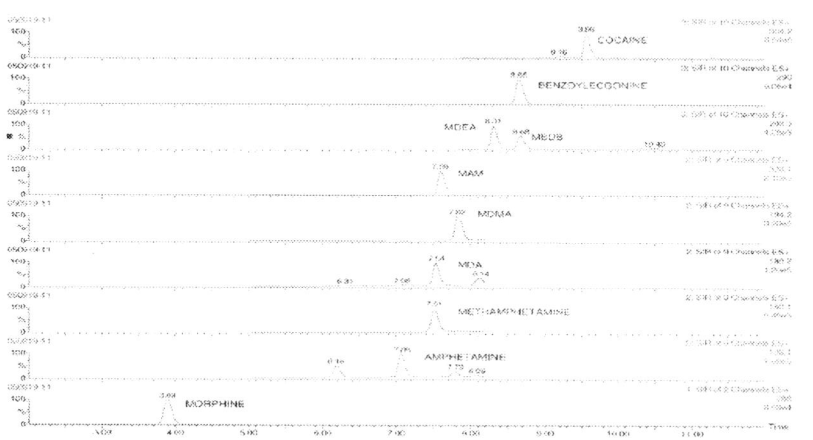

Source: Concheiro M, de Castro A, Quintela O, Lopez-Rivadulla M, Cruz A. Determination of drugs of abuse and their metabolites in human plasma by liquid chromatography-mass spectrometry: An application to 156 road fatalities. *Journal of Chromatography B-Analytical Technologies in the Biomedical and Life Sciences*. 2006;832,81-9. [37]

Figure 6. LC-MS quantitative ion chromatograms of plasma spiked at the 5 ng/mL level.

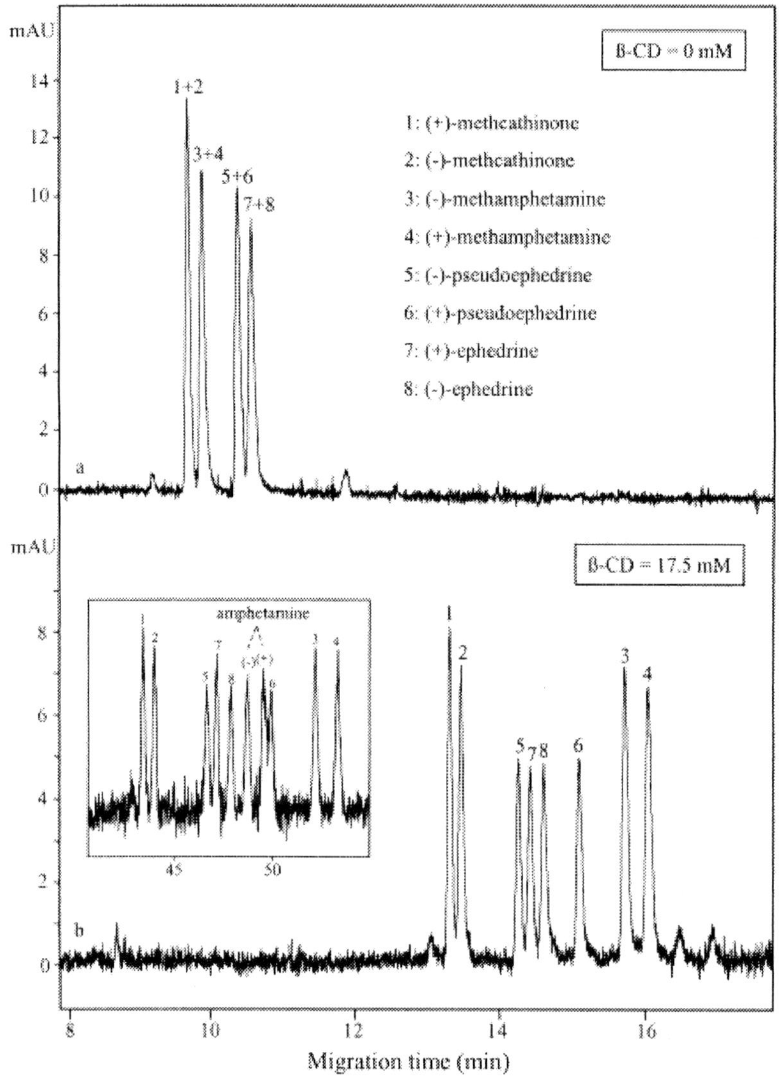

Source: Liau AS, Liu JT, Lin LC, Chiu YC, Shu YR, Tsai CC, Lin CH. Optimization of a simple method for the chiral separation of methamphetamine and related compounds in clandestine tablets and urine samples by β-cyclodextrin modified capillary electrophoresis: a complementary method to GC-MS. *Forensic Science International*. 2003;134,17-24. [63]

Figure 7. UV electropherograms of (±)-methamphetamine, (±)-methcathionone, (±)-ephedrine, and (±)-pseudoephedrine at 25 ppm concentration with and without the application of β-cyclodextrin.

METHOD SENSITIVITY

Accurate drug quantification is essential in providing evidence of illegal use and/or misuse. In the case of drugs that may impair judgment, *in vivo* concentrations can also help law enforcement understand the potential level of impairment. For the quantification of amphetamines, there are several methods that work down to the low ng/mL levels. Concheiro *et al.* presents an LC-ESI-MS/MS plasma method for measuring not only MAMP and MDMA, but also several other drugs of abuse, including cocaine and several opiate drugs [37]. This assay, while reporting only mediocre recovery (~50%), has an LOQ of 2 ng/mL [37]. Similar quantification limits, sample preparation (SPE), and analysis are reported for an almost identical set of drugs in saliva by Mortier *et al.* [64]. LC-MS/MS is not the only way to achieve sensitivity with amphetamine analysis; a 2006 paper by Hidvegi *et al.* reports quantification of MAMP, MDMA, and other amphetamine-type substances (ATS) by GC-EI-MS in serum at 5 ng/mL levels [52]. Scheidweiler & Huestis report similar LOQs for MAMP and MDMA using GC-EI-MS [6]. For hair analysis of MAMP and MDMA, one of the most sensitive methods is reported by Cheze *et al.* [65]. Using LC-ESI-MS/MS, this group measures 5 pg/mg of drug in hair samples as well as quantifying the same analytes in blood at 0.1 ng/mL levels [65]. Many labs are able to achieve quantification of $\leq$ 0.1 ng/mg of MAMP and/or MDMA in hair using LC-ESI-MS/MS, GC-EI-MS, and CE-MS [40,49,51,59,61,66,67].

MULTI-DRUG ANALYSIS

Many available MAMP methods are developed to also measure amphetamine. This is likely due to the fact that amphetamine is a major metabolite of MAMP, and is highly excreted in the urine unchanged [10]. The full metabolic scheme of MAMP is shown in the Figure 8 below [68]. While amphetamine is commonly thought of as the major metabolite of MAMP, Li *et al.* showed that the formation of this metabolite is much more enantioselective that the para-hydroxylated MAMP, thus suggesting that pOH-MAMP is a more suitable biomarker for MAMP use [68]. This metabolite, along with other ATS, has been quantitatively determined by Miki and colleagues from urine, blood, and hair using a unique on-column trifluoroacetylation derivatization and GC-MS [54]. Peters *et al.* used a heptofluorobutyric acid anhydride derivatization and GC-MS to quantify a similar set of compounds from plasma by GC-MS [69]. LC-MS has also been successfully applied to MAMP metabolite analysis, from blood [65,70,71], urine [5,53,65], and hair [65].

The majority of MAMP methods are developed to simultaneously measure MDMA. This is likely due to their common concurrent use within a group of drugs known as 'club drugs' which also includes gamma-hydroxybutyrate (GHB), ketamine (KET), and flunitrazepam (FLU). The most inclusive multi-drug method for screening of MAMP, MDMA, GHB, KET, FLU, as well as over 100 other drugs and metabolites, utilizes SPE, derivatization with N,O-bis-(trimethylsilyl) trifluoroacetamide (BSTFA) and trimethylchlorosilane (TCMS), and GC-EI-MS [72]. Some of these, including MAMP, are shown in Figure 9.

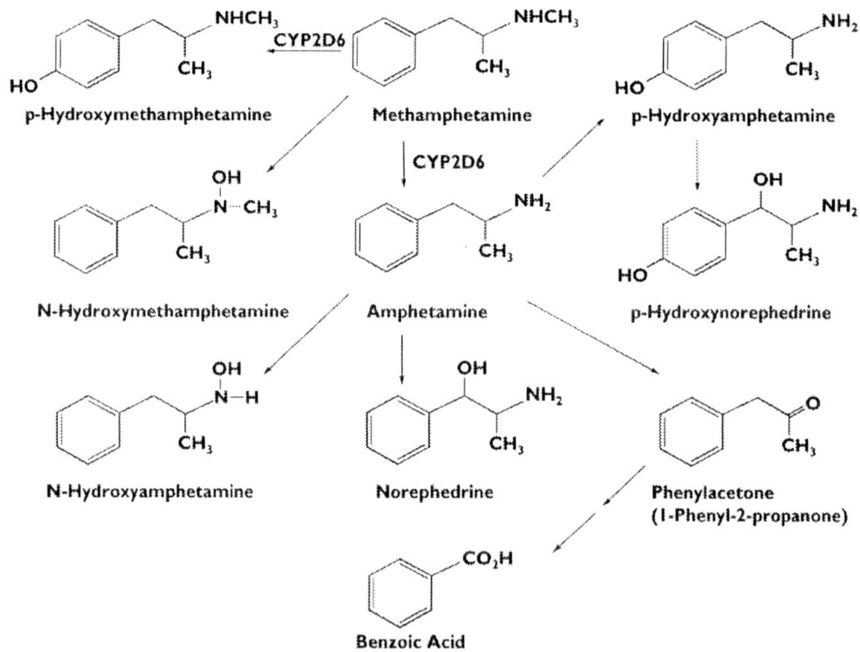

Source: Li L, Everhart T, Jacob P, Jones R. Stereoseletivity in the human metabolism of methamphetamine. *British Journal of Clinical Pharmacology*. 2010;69(2),187-92. [68]

Figure 8. Main metabolic pathways of methamphetamine in humans.

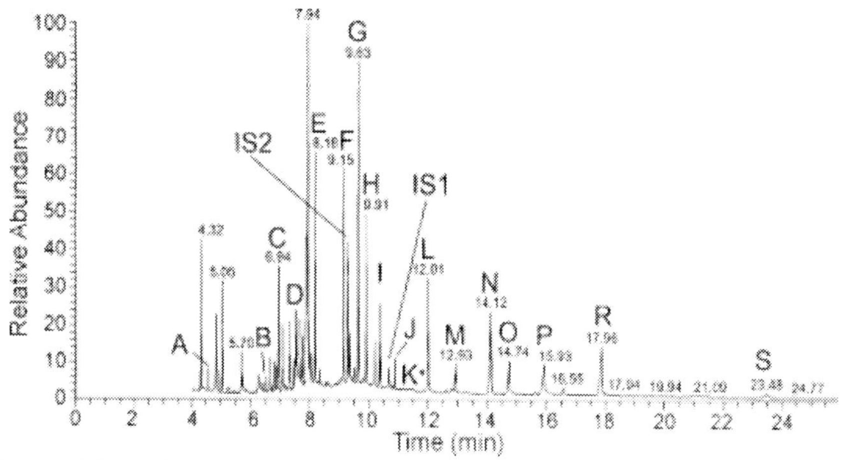

Source: Adamowicz P, Kala M. Simultaneous screening for and determination of 128 date-rape drugs in urine by gas chromatography-electron ionization-mass spectrometry. *Forensic Science International.* 2010;198,39-45. [72]

Figure 9. Total ion chromatogram (TIC) chromatogram of the extract of urine spiked with 18 analyzed compounds to the concentration of 10 μg/mL. A: methamphetamine, B: 4-methoxyamphetamine, C: 3,4-methylenedioxyamphetamine, D: pentobarbital, E: ketamine, F: brompheniramine, G: imipramine, H: promethazine, I: dosulepin, J: morphine, K: paroxetine (* <LOD), L: prazepam, M: flurazepam, N: clozapine, O: estazolam, P: zaleplon, R: thioridazine, S: buprenorphine, IS1: diazepam-D5, and IS2: methadone-D4.

A SPME-GC-MS method by Brown *et al.* includes quantifying MAMP, MDMA, GHB, and KET in urine with LOQs from 0.5 – 0.1 μg/mL [9]. The use of SPME as well as a derivatization scheme that works for every drug (hexylchloroformate and pyridine) facilitates this unique multi-drug assay. Lin *et al.* considered KET and MAMP from hair samples at relatively low levels (LOQ of 0.15 ng/mg) using micellular electrokinetic chromatography (MEKC), a type of CE separation [73]. Kuwayama *et al.* developed an LC-ESI-MS/MS method for quantification of MAMP, MDMA, KET, and other amphetamine-type substances (ATS) in plasma, urine, and bile using a simple protein precipitation sample preparation while maintaining respectable sensitivity (100 ng/mL) [5]. For the analysis of MAMP, MDMA, KET, and other drugs of abuse in hair, Wu *et al.* utilized a heptafluorobutyric acid anhydride heptafluorobutyric acid anhydride (HFBAA) derivatization coupled with SPE to prepare samples for GC-EI-MS [67]. Kim *et al.* was able to quantify MAMP, MDMA, KET and other ATS in fingernails at sub ng/mg levels using LLE, HFBAA derivatization and GC-EI-MS [48]. Finally, Sergi *et al.* worked with many of the same drugs as well as cocaine, phencyclidine, and tetrahydrocannabinol (THC) for quantification in plasma and saliva by LC-ESI-MS/MS using a very simple sample preparation of protein precipitation and filtration while managing to achieve LOQs for the drug analytes of < 2 ng/mL [23].

Conclusion

The analysis of methamphetamine in biological samples has received significant attention over the last decade. As use of this drug as well as its clandestine manufacture continues to rise, assays that have high sensitivity and specificity are needed for criminal investigations. In addition, legitimate uses of methamphetamine for treatment of ADD/ADHD and narcolepsy show need for such methods in the clinical pharmacokinetics and therapeutic drug monitoring fields. Immunoassays typically used in drug screening programs are plagued by cross reactivity with structural analogs, and this is especially true for amphetamines. For this reason, analyses that incorporate mass spectrometric detection have continued to prevail in this field, due to the specific fingerprint that the data provides. Fortunately, methamphetamine's structure lends itself to a wide variety of analytical possibilities, including capillary electrophoresis and liquid and gas chromatographic separations. Newer high resolution separation technologies such as ultra-high performance liquid chromatography are likely to become more prevalent in methamphetamine analysis as they become more common in forensic and drug research labs. Moving forward, the impact of multiple drug assays may continue to grow as labs search for more efficient ways to process samples as well as achieve detection of low concentrations that are often characteristic with drugs in biological samples and to capture relevant metabolite concentrations.

Acknowledgment

Parts of this chapter were previously published under the following reference: Brown SD, Melton TC. Trends in Bioanalytical Methods for Club Drugs: 2000-2010. *Biomedical Chromatography*. 2011;25,300-321. [74]

REFERENCES

[1] Jirovsky D, Lemr K, Sevcik J, Smysl B, Stransky Z. Methamphetamine – properties and analytical methods of enantiomer determination. *Forensic Science International.* 1998;96,61-70.

[2] Wu L, Schlenger W, Galvin D. Concurrent use of methamphetamine, MDMA, LSD, ketamine, GHB, and flunitrazepam among American youths. *Drug and Alcohol Dependence.* 2006;84,102-13.

[3] Barnes AJ, De Martinis BS, Gorelick DA, Goodwin RS, Kolbrich EA, Huestis MA. Disposition of MDMA and Metabolites in Human Sweat Following Controlled MDMA Administration. *Clinical Chemistry.* 2009;55,454-62.

[4] De Martinis BS, Barnes AJ, Scheidweiler KB, Huestis MA. Development and validation of a disk solid phase extraction and gas chromatography-mass spectrometry method for MDMA, MDA, HMMA, HMA, MDEA, methamphetamine and amphetamine in sweat. *Journal of Chroma-tography B-Analytical Technologies in the Biomedical and Life Sciences.* 2007;852,450-8.

[5] Kuwayama K, Inoue H, Kanamori T, Tsujikawa K, Miyaguchi H, Iwata YT, Miyauchi S, Kamo N. Analysis of amphetamine-type stimulants and their metabolites in plasma, urine and bile by liquid chromatography with a strong cation-exchange column-tandem mass spectrometry. *Journal of Chromatography B-Analytical Technologies in the Biomedical and Life Sciences.* 2008;867,78-83.

[6] Scheidweiler KB, Huestis MA. A validated gas chromatographic-electron impact ionization mass spectrometric method for methylenedioxy-methamphetamine (MDMA), methamphetamine and metabolites in oral fluid. *Journal of Chromatography B-Analytical Technologies in the Biomedical and Life Sciences.* 2006;835,90-9.

[7] Martyny JW, Arbuckle SL, McCammon Jr CS, Esswein EJ, Erb N, Van Dyke M. Chemical concentrations and contamination associated with clandestine methamphetamine laboratories. *Journal of Chemical Health and Safety.* 2007;14,40-52.

[8] Negrusz A, Gaensslen RE. Analytical developments in toxicological investigation of drug-facilitated sexual assault. *Analytical and Bio-analytical Chemistry.* 2003;376,1192-7.

[9] Brown SD, Rhodes DJ, Pritchard BJ. A validated SPME-GC-MS method for simultaneous quantification of club drugs in human urine. *Forensic Science International.* 2007;171,142-50.

[10] Dasgupta, A. A Health Educator's Guide to Understanding Drugs of Abuse Testing. Boston, MA: Jones and Bartlett Publishers; 2010.

[11] Meng PJ, Wang YY. Small volume liquid extraction of amphetamines in saliva. *Forensic Science International.* 2010;197,80-4.

[12] Molitor F, Truax S, Ruiz J, Sun R. Association of methamphetamine use during sex with risky sexual behaviors and HIV infection among non-injection drug users. *The Western Journal of Medicine.* 1998;168,93-7.

[13] Peters FT, Samyn N, Kraemer T, Riedel WJ, Maurer HH. Negative-ion chemical ionization gas chromatography-mass spectrometry assay for enantioselective measurement of amphetamines in oral fluid: Application to a controlled study with MDMA and driving under the influence cases. *Clinical Chemistry.* 2007;53,702-10.

[14] Navarro M, Pichini S, Farre M, Ortuno J, Roset PN, Segura J, de la Torre R. Usefulness of saliva for measurement of 3,4-methylenedioxy-methamphetamine and its metabolites: Correlation with plasma drug concentrations and effect of salivary pH. *Clinical Chemistry.* 2001;47,1788-95.

[15] Drummer OH. Review: Pharmacokinetics of illicit drugs in oral fluid. *Forensic Science International.* 2005;150,133-42.

[16] De Paoli G, Bell S. A rapid GC-MS determination of gamma-hydroxybutyrate in saliva. *Journal of Analytical Toxicology.* 2008; 32,298-302.

[17] Joya X, Pujadas M, Falcon M, Civit E, Garcia-Algar O, Vall O, Pichini S, Luna A, de la Torre R. Gas chromatography-mass spectrometry assay for the simultaneous quantification of drugs of abuse in human placenta at 12th week of gestation. *Forensic Science International.* 2010;196,38-42.

[18] Kelly T, Gray TR, Huestis MA. Development and validation of a liquid chromatography-atmospheric pressure chemical ionization-tandem mass spectrometry method for simultaneous analysis of 10 amphetamine-, methamphetamine- and 3,4-methylenedioxymethamphetamine-related (MDMA) analytes in human meconium. *Journal of Chromatography B-Analytical Technologies in the Biomedical and Life Sciences.* 2008; 867,194-204.

[19] Scheidweiler KB, Barnes AJ, Huestis MA. A validated gas chromatographic-electron impact ionization mass spectrometric method for methamphetamine, methylenedioxymethamphetamine (MDMA), and metabolites in mouse plasma and brain. *Journal of Chromatography B-*

Analytical Technologies in the Biomedical and Life Sciences. 2008;876,266-76.

[20] Deveaux M, Cheze M, Pepin G. The role of liquid chromatography-tandem mass Spectrometry (LC-MS/MS) to test blood and urine samples for the toxicological investigation of drug-facilitated crimes. *Therapeutic Drug Monitoring.* 2008;30,225-8.

[21] Sasaki T. Forensic toxicology widens net for drugs of abuse: the rise of LC/MS/MS for toxicology testing. *Forensic Magazine.* 2007;October/November.

[22] Huang Z, Zhang S. Confirmation of amphetamine, methamphetamine, MDA, and MDMA in urine samples using disk solid-phase extraction and gas-chromatography -mass spectrometry after immunoassay screening. *Journal of Chrmoatography B.* 2003;792,241-7.

[23] Sergi M, Bafile E, Compagnone D, Curini R, D'Ascenzo G, Romolo FS. Multiclass analysis of illicit drugs in plasma and oral fluids by LC-MS/MS. *Analytical and Bioanalytical Chemistry.* 2009;393,709-18.

[24] Shima N, Kamata H, Katagi M, Tsuchihashi H, Sakuma T, Nemoto N. Direct determination of glucuronide and sulfate of 4-hydroxy-3-methoxymethamphetamine, the main metabolite of MDMA, in human urine. *Journal of Chromatography B-Analytical Technologies in the Biomedical and Life Sciences.* 2007;857,123-9.

[25] Vlase L, Popa DS, Loghin F, Leucuta SE. High-throughput toxicological analysis of Methamphetamine, MDA and MDMA from human plasma by LC-MS/MS. *Romanian Journal of Legal Medicine.* 2009;17,213-20.

[26] Kato N, Fujita S, Ohta H, Fukuba M, Toriba A, Hayakawa K. Thin Layer Chromatography/Fluorescence Detection of 3,4-Methylenedioxy-Methamphetamine and Related Compounds. *Journal of Forensic Sciences.* 2008;53,1367-71.

[27] Chen CY, Lee MR, Cheng FC, Wu GJ. Determination of ketamine and metabolites in urine by liquid chromatography-mass spectrometry. *Talanta.* 2007;72,1217-22.

[28] Pawliszyn J. Solid Phase Microextraction Theory and Practice. New York, NY: Wiley-VCH; 1997.

[29] Pan L, Pawliszyn J. Derivatization/solid-phase microextraction: new approach to polar analytes. *Analytical Chemistry.* 1997;69,196-205.

[30] Chia KJ, Huang SD. Simultaneous derivatization and extraction of amphetamine-like drugs in urine with headspace solid-phase microextraction followed by gas chromatography-mass spectrometry. *Analytica Chimica Acta.* 2005;539,49-54.

[31] Bugey A, Staub C. Rapid analysis of benzodiazepines in whole blood by high-performance liquid chromatography: use of a monolithic column. *Journal of Pharmaceutical and Biomedical Analysis.* 2004;35,555-62.

[32] Darius J, Banditt P. Validated method for the therapeutic drug monitoring of flunitrazepam in human serum using liquid chromatography-atmospheric pressure chemical ionization tandem mass spectrometry with an ion trap detector. *Journal of Chromatography B.* 2000;738,437-41.

[33] Hegstad S, Oiestad EL, Johansen U, Christophersen AS. Determination of benzodiazepines in human urine using solid-phase extraction and high-performance liquid chromatography-electrospray ionization tandem mass spectrometry. *Journal of Analytical Toxicology.* 2006;30,31-7.

[34] Huang MK, Liu CR, Huang SD. One step and highly sensitive headspace solid-phase microextraction sample preparation approach for the analysis of methamphetamine and amphetamine in human urine. *Analyst.* 2002;127,1203-6.

[35] Kollroser M, Schober C. Simultaneous analysis of flunitrazepam and its major metabolites in human plasma by high performance liquid chromatography tandem mass spectrometry. *Journal of Pharmaceutical and Biomedical Analysis.* 2002;28,1173-82.

[36] Fernandez M, Laloup M, Wood M, De Boeck G, Lopez-Rivadulla M, Wallemacq P, Samyn N. Liquid chromatography-tandem mass spectrometry method for the simultaneous analysis of multiple hallucinogens, chlorpheniramine, ketamine, ritalinic acid, and metabolites, in urine. *Journal of Analytical Toxicology.* 2007;31,497-504.

[37] Concheiro M, de Castro A, Quintela O, Lopez-Rivadulla M, Cruz A. Determination of drugs of abuse and their metabolites in human plasma by liquid chromatography-mass spectrometry - An application to 156 road fatalities. *Journal of Chromatography B-Analytical Technologies in the Biomedical and Life Sciences.* 2006;832,81-9.

[38] Concheiro M, Simoes SMD, Quintela O, de Castro A, Dias MJR, Cruz A, Lopez-Rivadulla M. Fast LC-MS/MS method for the determination of amphetamine, methamphetamine, MDA, MDMA, MDEA, MBDB and PMA in urine. *Forensic Science International.* 2007;171,44-51.

[39] Villamor JL, Bermejo AM, Fernandez P, Tabernero MJ. GC-MS determination of amphetamines in human urine. *Analytical Letters.* 2005;38,781-90.

[40] Gottardo R, Bortolotti F, De Paoli G, Pascali JP, Miksik I, Tagliaro F. Hair analysis for illicit drugs by using capillary zone electrophoresis-electrospray ionization-ion trap mass spectrometry. *Journal of Chromatography A.* 2007;1159,185-9.

[41] Apollonio L, Pianca D, Whittall I, Kyd J, Maher W. A comparison of atmospheric pressure chemical ionization and electrospray ionization in testing for amphetamine-type substances and ketamine using ultra-performance liquid chromatography/mass spectrometry. *Rapid Communications in Mass Spectrometry.* 2006;20,2777-80.

[42] Apollonio LG, Pianca DJ, Whittall IR, Maher WA, Kyd JM. A demonstration of the use of ultra-performance liquid chromatography-mass spectrometry [UPLC/MS] in the determination of amphetamine-type substances and ketamine for forensic and toxicological analysis. *Journal of Chromatography B-Analytical Technologies in the Biomedical and Life Sciences.* 2006;836,111-5.

[43] Bergo PLD, Correa JM, Nagem TJ, Augusti R, Nascentes CC. Simultaneous Quantification of Amphetamines and Ephedrines in Urine by GC/MS using Analytical-Grade Acetic Anhydride/Pyridine as Derivatizing Reagents: a Suitable Approach to Reduce Costs of Routine Analyses. *Journal of the Brazilian Chemical Society.* 2009;20,348-59.

[44] Watanabe K, Okamoto N, Yamagishi I, Nozawa H, Ishii A, Suzuki O. Simple analysis of amphetamines in human whole blood and urine by headspace capillary gas chromatography with large volume injection. *Chromatographia.* 2003;58,455-8.

[45] Ye NS, Gu XX, Wang JF, Sun HF, Li WJ, Zhang YQ. MAE-GC Determination of Methamphetamine, 3,4-Methylenedioxyamphetamine and 3,4-Methylenedioxymethamphetamine in Human Urine. *Chromatographia.* 2009;69,933-9.

[46] Matuszewski BK, Constanzer ML, Chavez-Eng CM. Matrix Effect in Quantitative LC/MS/MS Analyses of Biological Fluids: A Method for Determination of Finasteride in Human Plasma at Picogram Per Milliliter Concentrations. *Analytical Chemistry.* 1998;70,882-9.

[47] King R, Bonfiglio R, Fernandez-Metzler C, Miller-Stein C, Olah T. Mechanistic investigation of ionization suppression in electrospray ionization. *Journal of the American Society for Mass Spectrometry.* 2000;11,942-50.

[48] Kim JY, Shin SH, In MK. Determination of amphetamine-type stimulants, ketamine and metabolites in fingernails by gas chromate-

graphy-mass spectrometry. *Forensic Science International.* 2010; 194,108-14.

[49] Kim JY, Shin SH, Lee JI, In MK. Rapid and simple determination of psychotropic phenylalkylamine derivatives in human hair by gas chromatography-mass spectrometry using micro-pulverized extraction. *Forensic Science International.* 2010;196,43-50.

[50] Jurado C, Gimenez MP, Soriano T, Menendez M, Repetto M. Rapid analysis of amphetamine, methamphetamine, MDA, and MDMA in urine using solid-phase microextraction, direct on-fiber derivatization, and analysis by GC-MS. *Journal of Analytical Toxicology.* 2000;24,11-6.

[51] Kim JY, Jung KS, Kim MK, Il Lee J, In MK. Simultaneous determination of psychotropic phenylalkylamine derivatives in human hair by gas chromatography/mass spectrometry. *Rapid Communications in Mass Spectrometry.* 2007;21,1705-20.

[52] Hidvegi E, Fabian P, Hideg Z, Somogyi G. GC-MS determination of amphetamines in serum using on-line trifluoroacetylation. *Forensic Science International.* 2006;161,119-23.

[53] Kim JY, Cheong JC, Kim MK, Lee JI, In MK. Simultaneous determination of amphetamine-type stimulants and cannabinoids in fingernails by gas chromatography-mass spectrometry. *Archives of Pharmacal Research.* 2008;31,805-13.

[54] Miki A, Katagi M, Zaitsu K, Nishioka H, Tsuchihashi H. Development of a two-step injector for GC-MS with on-column derivatization, and its application to the determination of amphetamine-type stimulants (ATS) in biological specimens. *Journal of Chromatography B-Analytical Technologies in the Biomedical and Life Sciences.* 2008;865,25-32.

[55] Martins LF, Yegles M, Chung H, Wennig R. Sensitive, rapid and validated gas chromatography/negative ion chemical ionization-mass spectrometry assay including derivatization with a novel chiral agent for the enantioselective quantification of amphetamine-type stimulants in hair. *Journal of Chromatography B-Analytical Technologies in the Biomedical and Life Sciences.* 2006;842,98-105.

[56] Bugamelli F, Mandrioli R, Cavallini A, Baccini C, Conti M, Raggi MA. Determination of amphetamines in human urine by liquid chromatography with fluorimetric detection using a solid-phase extraction procedure. *Journal of Separation Science.* 2006;29,2322-9.

[57] Chafer-Pericas C, Campins-Falco P, Herraez-Hernandez R. Application of solid-phase microextraction combined with derivatization to the

determination of amphetamines by liquid chromatography. *Analytical Biochemistry*. 2004;333,328-35.

[58] Kaddoumi A, Kikura-Hanajiri R, Nakashima K. High-performance liquid chromatography with fluorescence detection for the simultaneous determination of 3,4-methylenedioxymethamphetamine, methamphetamine and their metabolites in human hair using DIB-Cl as a label. *Biomedical Chromatography*. 2004;18,202-4.

[59] Nakamura S, Tomita M, Wada M, Chung HS, Kuroda N, Nakashima K. Quantification of MDMA and MDA in abusers' hair samples by semi-micro column HPLC with fluorescence detection. *Biomedical Chromatography*. 2006;20,622-7.

[60] Wada M, Nakamura S, Tomita M, Nakashima MN, Nakashima K. Determination of MDMA and MDA in rat urine by semi-micro column HPLC-fluorescence detection with DBD-F and their monitoring after MDMA administration to rat. *Luminescence*. 2005;20,210-5.

[61] Li XQ, Uboh CE, Soma LR, Guan FY, You YW, Kahler MC, Judy JA, Liu Y, Chen JW. Simultaneous separation and confirmation of amphetamine and related drugs in equine plasma by non-aqueous capillary-electrophoresis-tandem mass spectrometry. *Drug Testing and Analysis*. 2010;2,70-81.

[62] Jen HP, Tsai YC, Su HL, Hsieh YZ. On-line preconcentration and determination of ketamine and norketamine by micellar electrokinetic chromatography - Complementary method to gas chromatography/mass spectrometry. *Journal of Chromatography A*. 2006;1111,159-65.

[63] Liau AS, Liu JT, Lin LC, Chiu YC, Shu YR, Tsai CC, Lin CH. Optimization of a simple method for the chiral separation of methamphetamine and related compounds in clandestine tablets and urine samples by b-cyclodextrin modified capillary electrophoresis: a complementary method to GC-MS. *Forensic Science International*. 2003;134,17-24.

[64] Mortier KA, Maudens KE, Lambert WE, Clauwaert KM, Van Bocxlaer JF, Deforce DL, Van Peteghem CH, De Leenheer AP. Simultaneous, quantitative determination of opiates, amphetamines, cocaine and benzoylecgonine in oral fluid by liquid chromatography quadrupole-time-of-flight mass spectrometry. *Journal of Chromatography B-Analytical Technologies in the Biomedical and Life Sciences*. 2002;779,321-30.

[65] Cheze M, Deveaux M, Martin C, Lhermitte M, Pepin G. Simultaneous analysis of six amphetamines and analogues in hair, blood and urine by

LC-ESI-MS/MS Application to the determination of MDMA after low Ecstasy intake. *Forensic Science International.* 2007;170,100-4.

[66] Musshoff F, Junker HP, Lachenmeier DW, Kroener L, Madea B. Fully automated determination of amphetamines and synthetic designer drugs in hair samples using headspace solid-phase microextraction and gas chromatography-mass spectrometry. *Journal of Chromatographic Science.* 2002;40,359-64.

[67] Wu YH, Lin KL, Chen SC, Chang YZ. Simultaneous quantitative determination of amphetamines, ketamine, opiates and metabolites in human hair by gas chromatography/mass spectrometry. *Rapid Communications in Mass Spectrometry.* 2008;22,887-97.

[68] Li L, Everhart T, Jacob P, Jones R. Stereoseletivity in the human metabolism of methamphetamine. *British Journal of Clinical Pharmacology.* 2010;69,187-92.

[69] Peters FT, Schaefer S, Staack RF, Kraemer T, Maurer HH. Screening for and validated quantification of amphetamines and of amphetamine- and piperazine-derived designer drugs in human blood plasma by gas chromatography/mass spectrometry. *Journal of Mass Spectrometry.* 2003;38,659-76.

[70] Bjork MK, Nielsen MKK, Markussen LO, Klinke HB, Linnet K. Determination of 19 drugs of abuse and metabolites in whole blood by high-performance liquid chromatography-tandem mass spectrometry. *Analytical and Bioanalytical Chemistry.* 2010;396,2393-401.

[71] Shima N, Katagi M, Kamata H, Zaitsu K, Kamata T, Miki A, Tsuchihashi H, Sakuma T, Nemoto N. Conjugates of p-hydroxy-methamphetamine and 4-hydroxy-3-methoxymethamphetamine in blood obtained from methamphetamine and 3,4-methylenedioxy-methamphetamine users: analysis by LC-MS-MS. *Forensic Toxicology.* 2008;26,58-65.

[72] Adamowicz P, Kala M. Simultaneous screening for and determination of 128 date-rape drugs in urine by gas chromatography-electron ionization-mass spectrometry. *Forensic Science International.* 2010;1980,39-45.

[73] Lin YH, Lee MR, Lee RJ, Ko WK, Wu SM. Hair analysis for methamphetamine, ketamine, morphine and codeine by cation-selective exhaustive injection and sweeping micellar electrokinetic chromatography. *Journal of Chromatography A.* 2007;1145,234-40.

[74] Brown SD, Melton TC. Trends in Bioanalytical Methods for Club Drugs: 2000-2010. *Biomedical Chromatography.* 2011;25,300-321.

In: Methamphetamines
Editors: J. Ornoy and X. He

ISBN: 978-1-62100-244-4

Chapter 5

ISOLIQUIRITIGENIN, A LICORICE FLAVONOID, INHIBITS METHAMPHETAMINE-INDUCED HYPERLOCOMOTION BUT NOT STEREOTYPY OR CONDITIONED PLACE PREFERENCE IN MICE

Nobue Kitanaka[1], Junichi Kitanaka[1,*], Hiroki Minami,[1,†] Masayuki Okamoto,[1,†] Tomohiro Tatsuta,[2] Yoshio Morita,[3] Koh-ichi Tanaka,[4] Nobuyoshi Nishiyama,[4] and Motohiko Takemura[1]

[1]Department of Pharmacology, Hyogo College of Medicine, Nishinomiya, Hyogo, Japan

[2]Ibogawa Hospital Furuhashikai Medical Corporation, Hyogo 671-1688, Japan

[3]Faculty of Nursing, Baika Women's University, Osaka, Japan

[4]Division of Pharmacology, Department of Pharmacy, School of Pharmacy, Hyogo University of Health Sciences, 1-3-6 Minatojima, Chuo-ku, Kobe, Hyogo, Japan

[*] Corresponding author. Department of Pharmacology, Hyogo College of Medicine, 1-1 Mukogawa-cho, Nishinomiya, Hyogo 663-8501, Japan. Phone: +81 798 456333; Fax: +81 798 456332; E-mail: kitanaka-hyg@umin.net.

[†] These authors contributed equally to this study as medical students participating in an orientation course for medical sciences (2010) held at the Department of Pharmacology, Hyogo College of Medicine.

ABSTRACT

We investigated whether pretreatment with isoliquiritigenin (ISL), an anti-oxidant flavonoid obtained from *Glycyrrhizae* species, affected methamphetamine (METH)-induced hyperlocomotion, conditioned place preference (CPP), and stereotypy in mice. Pretreatment of male ICR mice with ISL (20 mg/kg, i.p.) significantly inhibited METH (1 mg/kg, i.p.)-induced hyperlocomotion compared with that of vehicle-pretreated subjects, but there were no significant alterations in the tissue levels of monoamines and their metabolites in the cerebral cortex, the region of striatum and nucleus accumbens, and the region of thalamus and hypothalamus between mice with and without ISL pretreatment. Mice treated with ISL prior to METH (0.5 mg/kg) preconditioning showed a significant METH-induced CPP, similar to that observed in mice treated with vehicle prior to METH preconditioning. The total incidence of METH (10 mg/kg)-induced stereotypy was unaffected by pretreatment with ISL. These observations suggest that ISL selectively inhibits METH-induced hyperlocomotion in mice.

Keywords: Methamphetamine; isoliquiritigenin; hyperlocomotion; stereotypy; conditioned place preference; monoamine metabolism

ABBREVIATIONS

ANOVA	analysis of variance;
CPP	conditioned place preference;
DOPAC	3:4-dihydroxyphenylacetic acid;
DA	dopamine;
5-HIAA	5-hydroxyindolacetic acid;
HPLC	high-performance liquid chromatography;
5-HT	5-hydroxytryptamine (serotonin);
HVA	homovanillic acid;
i.p.	intraperitoneally;
ISL	isoliquiritigenin;
METH	methamphetamine;

MHPG	3-methoxy-4-hydroxyphenylglycol;
3-MT	3-methoxytyramine;
NAc	nucleus accumbens;
N.D.	not detected;
NE	norepinephrine;
SEM	standard error of the mean.

INTRODUCTION

Methamphetamine (METH) is one of the most powerful addictive psychostimulants recognized worldwide (National Institute on Drug Abuse, 2004), and is a popular recreational drug of abuse in Japan as a third epidemic of METH abuse (Ujike and Sato, 2004). It is important to establish a medication for METH-induced pathologies including euphoria, increased respiration, hyperthermia, enhanced body movements, and amphetamine psychosis, although successful treatments for METH abusers remain elusive (Srisurapanont et al., 2001; Kantak, 2003).

METH targets in subcellular components include the cocaine-sensitive dopamine transporter (DAT), the vesicular monoamine transporter-2 (VMAT-2), and the monoamine oxidase (MAO) isozymes (Seiden et al., 1993; Sulzer et al., 2005). Interacting with these subcellular components, METH causes a massive release of monoamines, mainly dopamine (DA), from the presynaptic terminal into the synaptic cleft in the brain (Di Chiara and Imperato, 1988). The excessive release of DA has been believed to overactivate DAnergic pathways such as mesolimbic and nigrostriatal pathways, resulting in particular pathologies. The DA hypothesis has been supported by evidence that some of these pathologies can be treated with DA receptor antagonists such as haloperidol (Mori et al., 2004; Tada et al., 2004) with an extrapyramidal side effect under high-dosing of the DA receptor antagonists. Search for novel compounds with pharmacological properties different from classical DA receptor antagonists is one promising approach for the development of a treatment for METH abusers, avoiding the side effects of classical DA receptor antagonists effectively.

Isoliquiritigenin (ISL; 2’,4’,4-trihydroxychalcone), a flavonoid chalcone found in licorice roots and other plants including shallots, has been reported to have anti-oxidant and anti-tumor activities including suppression of both proliferation of tumor cells and tumor-induced angiogenesis (Yamamoto et al., 1991; Chin et al., 2007; Sun et al., 2010). Recently, the effects of ISL on psychostimulant-induced biological alterations have also been reported. For instance, pretreatment with ISL attenuated cocaine-induced extracellular DA release in the nucleus accumbens of the rat (Jang et al., 2008) and METH-induced loss of striatal DAT-like and tyrosine hydroxylase-like immune-reactivity in mice (Lee et al., 2009). These observations suggest that pretreatment with ISL inhibits METH-induced behavioral alterations. Regarding this point, Jeon et al. (2008) reported that pretreatment of rats with ISL inhibited cocaine-induced hyperlocomotion.

In the present study, the effects of ISL on METH-induced hyper-locomotion, conditioned place preference (CPP), and stereotypy in mice were investigated in order to shed light on the possibility of using ISL for treatment of METH-induced mental and physical illness.

Materials and Methods

Subjects

Male ICR mice (10-13 weeks old; Japan SLC, Shizuoka, Japan) were housed in groups of eight (cage size: 37 x 22 x 15 cm) in a temperature- (22 ± 2°C) and humidity-controlled (50 ± 10%) environment under a 12 h light/dark cycle (lights on at 07:00) with food and water available *ad libitum* except during testing. Animal handling and care were conducted according to the *Guide for the Care and Use of Laboratory Animals* (7th edition, Institute of Laboratory Animal Resources-National Research Council, National Academy Press 1996), and all experiments were reviewed and approved by our Institutional Animal Research Committee. Mice were used only once (body weight on experimental day: 36-47 g, n = 82 total) after at least one week of habituation in the facility.

Reagents

METH hydrochloride was purchased from Dainippon Sumitomo Pharma Co., Ltd. (Osaka, Japan). ISL ((*E*)-1-(2,4-dihydroxyphenyl)-3-(4-hydroxy-phenyl)-2-propen-1-one) was purchased from Sigma-Aldrich (St. Louis, MO,

USA). All other chemicals used were of the highest purity commercially available. The doses of drugs refer to the weight of salt. METH was dissolved in sterile saline. ISL was dissolved in vehicle (Tween 80:polyethylene glycol 200:ethanol:water = 7:1:1:1, by volume) and sonicated for 5 min. Drug solutions were prepared in such a way that the necessary dose could be injected in a volume of 0.1 ml/10 g of body weight by an i.p. route (METH) or in a volume of 0.05 ml/10 g of body weight by an i.p. route (ISL).

Treatment Protocol and Measurement

Effect of ISL on METH-induced Hyperlocomotion

Mice were weighed, divided randomly into two groups ($n = 7$ per group), and treated with 20 mg/kg ISL or vehicle. The dose of ISL was chosen on the basis of reports in the literature (Jang et al., 2008; Jeon et al., 2008). After the pretreatment injection, all mice were placed in the test box for measurement of locomotor activity for 30 min. Thirty minutes later, all mice were injected with 1 mg/kg METH, and were placed in the test box for measurement of locomotor activity for 1 h. Locomotor activity was measured in a transparent acrylic test box (30 x 30 x 35 cm) with approximately 25 g of fresh wood chips spread on the floor of the chamber using an Animex Auto apparatus (System MK-110; Muromachi Kikai Co., Ltd., Tokyo, Japan) in a quiet room as described previously (Kitanaka et al., 2003). The apparatus detects changes in electrical capacitance (oscillation frequency) in an LC oscillator circuit system under the floor of the apparatus as an animal moves horizontally in an electric field. In this set of experiments, the sensitivity parameter was set at 580 (Kitanaka et al., 2003). Under this criterion, the count of oscillation frequency parallels the degree of horizontal locomotion. The acrylic test boxes were cleaned and wiped dry between sessions for each animal. All experiments were conducted between 9:00 and 15:30.

Effect of ISL on Tissue Levels of Monoamines and their Metabolites in Brain Regions of Mice Challenged with METH

Mice were weighed, divided randomly into two groups ($n = 6$ per group), and treated with 20 mg/kg ISL or vehicle. After the pretreatment injection, all mice were placed in the test apparatus for 30 min (but without measurement of locomotor activity). Thirty minutes later, all mice were injected with 1 mg/kg METH, and were placed in the test apparatus (but without measurement of locomotor activity). Mice were sacrificed by cervical dislocation and decapitation 40 min after the METH challenge. The brains were immediately removed, and the cerebral cortices, regions of the striata and accumbens, and regions of the thalami and hypothalami were isolated, weighed, and frozen in liquid nitrogen until assay by HPLC.

The tissue levels of monoamines and metabolites were quantified by HPLC with electrochemical detection as described previously (Kitanaka et al., 2003). Each frozen brain sample was homogenized with a Teflon/glass homogenizer in 5 volumes (w/v) of ice-cold 0.1 N perchloric acid with 30 μM Na_2 EDTA containing 3,4-dihydroxybenzylamine hydrobromide and isoproterenol as internal standards for the catechols and indoles, respectively. The homogenates were centrifuged at 10,000 x *g* for 10 min at 4°C, and the supernatants were filtered through a 0.20-μm membrane filter (Millipore Co., Bedford, MA, USA). The filtrates (10 μl) were injected directly into an HPLC system (system controller: model SCL-10A; auto-injector: model SIL-10A; pump: model LC-10AD; Shimadzu Co., Kyoto, Japan) equipped with a reversed-phase ODS-column (MCM column 150; 4.6 x 150 mm; MC Medical, Inc., Osaka, Japan) and an electrochemical detector (Coulochem Model 5100A, ESA, Inc., Chelmsford, MA, USA). The column temperature was maintained at 24°C, and the detector potentials were set at +0.40 V, +0.05 V, and -0.30 V for the conditioning cell and detectors 1 and 2, respectively. The mobile phase was a 1000:35.2:85.8 (v/v) mixture of a buffer (50 mM Na_2HPO_4, 50 mM citric acid, 4.4 mM 1-heptanesulfonic acid, and 0.1 mM Na_2EDTA, pH 3.0), acetonitrile, and methanol, and the flow rate was set at 0.9 ml/min.

Effect of ISL on METH-induced CPP

The place preference apparatus was developed at Muromachi Kikai Co., Ltd. (Tokyo, Japan) using Supermex® sensors (Kitanaka et al., 2006). The infrared pyroelectric sensors were originally developed to measure horizontal locomotor activity by detecting the body heat of an animal (Kitanaka et al., 2003). The CPP boxes were made of acrylic resin, with two main compartments of 24.3 x 15.6 x 21.3 cm, divided by a removable barrier with a doorway (8.0 x 6.0 cm). A solid barrier without a doorway was used to confine animals to a given side of the compartment. Two sensors were positioned on the top cover of each compartment of the CPP box. The data collected from the sensors concerned horizontal locomotor activity as well as the time spent in each compartment. When the animal entered and stayed in an overlapping detection area of the two sensors (1.8 cm each from the border of the two compartment floors), the animal was defined as being in a "neutral" position. The collected data were analyzed using a newly developed program (CompACT CPP for Windows, version 1.40, Muromachi Kikai, Co., Ltd.) running on a PC computer. The compartments had different visual and textural cues (one was black with a smooth floor and the other was white with 5 g of fresh wood-chips on a smooth floor). All compartments were cleaned and wiped dry between the sessions for each animal.

On day 1, mice were weighed (n = 24) and placed in CPP boxes for preconditioning with no injection; the mice were placed into the neutral position and then allowed free access to the two compartments for 10 min. The compartment in which the mice stayed for a shorter time was defined as the conditioning compartment. The definition was based on an individual animal (a biased design). Mice were then randomly assigned to either the METH/saline conditioning group or saline/saline control group (n = 12 each). The second phase consisted of six days (three METH/saline or three saline/saline pairings) of conditioning. Two hours after lights on, six mice in each group received injections of ISL (20 mg/kg) or vehicle once per day for six consecutive days, and were then returned to their home cages. On days 3, 5, and 7, 30 min after ISL/vehicle pretreatment, the mice received injections of saline or METH (0.5 mg/kg) in the conditioning compartment determined on day 1, and were then confined to the conditioning compartment for 20 min. On days 4, 6, and 8, all mice were injected with saline and immediately confined to the opposite compartment for 20 min. Control mice therefore received saline in both compartments once per day for six consecutive days in this conditioning phase. On day 9 (post-conditioning day), mice were placed in the neutral position and then allowed 10 min with free access to the two compartments. Data regarding time spent in each compartment and locomotor activity (number of signal changes in sensor elements) were recorded using the computerized system (Kitanaka et al., 2006). The difference in time spent in the conditioning compartment between post-conditioning (day 9) and preconditioning (day 1) sessions for each treatment was analyzed as a CPP index. The experimental room was kept quiet, and all experiments were conducted between 9:00 and 15:00. All mice maintained or gained body weight during the experimental period (data not shown).

Effect of ISL on METH-induced Stereotypy and Horizontal Locomotion

Mice were weighed and divided randomly into four groups (n = 8 per group). Subjects were treated with 10 mg/kg METH 30 min after ISL or vehicle injection. After the challenge injection, all mice were placed in the testing apparatus for measurement of locomotor activity and rating of stereotypic behavior for 1 h as described below.

Test subjects were placed in a transparent acrylic test box for measurement of locomotor activity and observed for stereotypy for 1 h after drug administration by trained observers unaware of the treatments. Behavior was assessed in 30-s intervals, and the predominant behavior observed during each interval was recorded. Since individual stereotypical behaviors were unchanged for long periods (>30 s) after drug treatment, it was possible to record the observations by hand. The behaviors scored were inactive (awake and inactive, or sleeping), ambulating, rearing, persistent locomotion, head bobbing (up-and-down movements of the head), continuous sniffing, circling, and continuous nail and/or wood-chip biting or licking, according to a method described previously (Kitanaka et al., 2010). Ambulating, rearing, and persistent locomotion were considered locomotor and exploratory behaviors, and the last four categories were considered stereotypies. Persistent locomotion was not classified as a stereotypy because the mice scored as having "persistent locomotion" showed horizontal locomotor activity less than or equal to that displayed by mice showing "hyperlocomotion" (which is not generally defined as a stereotypy) measured by Animex Auto (Kitanaka et al., 2005, 2010). The cumulative number of intervals within each 5 min period in which stereotypies were rated is shown as a time course below (maximal value = 10).

Statistics

Data are presented as mean ± the standard error of the mean (SEM). Statistical analysis was performed using mixed factor analysis of variance (ANOVA) with or without repeated measures followed by Bonferroni/Dunn *post hoc* tests (Statview 5.0 for Apple Macintosh, SAS Institute, Inc., Cary, NC, USA). For the HPLC analysis, data were analyzed by Fisher's PLSD tests when ANOVA showed significant main effect(s). $P < 0.05$ was considered statistically significant.

RESULTS

Effect of ISL on METH-Induced Hyperlocomotion

Figure 1 shows METH-induced hyperlocomotion and the effect of ISL pretreatment on mice. A repeated-measures ANOVA (Pretreatment x Time) applied to the data represented in Figure 1 (Time = -30-0 min after challenge) revealed a significant main effect of Time ($F(5,72) = 2.505$, $P < 0.05$), but no significant main effect of Pretreatment ($F(1,72) = 0.224$, $P = 0.6448$) and Pretreatment x Time interaction ($F(5,72) = 1.525$, $P = 0.1955$). Bonferroni-corrected pairwise comparisons found that locomotor activity at time 0 was significantly decreased compared with those observed during the period between time –30 and -15 ($P < 0.05$), probably due to habituation to the measurement environment.

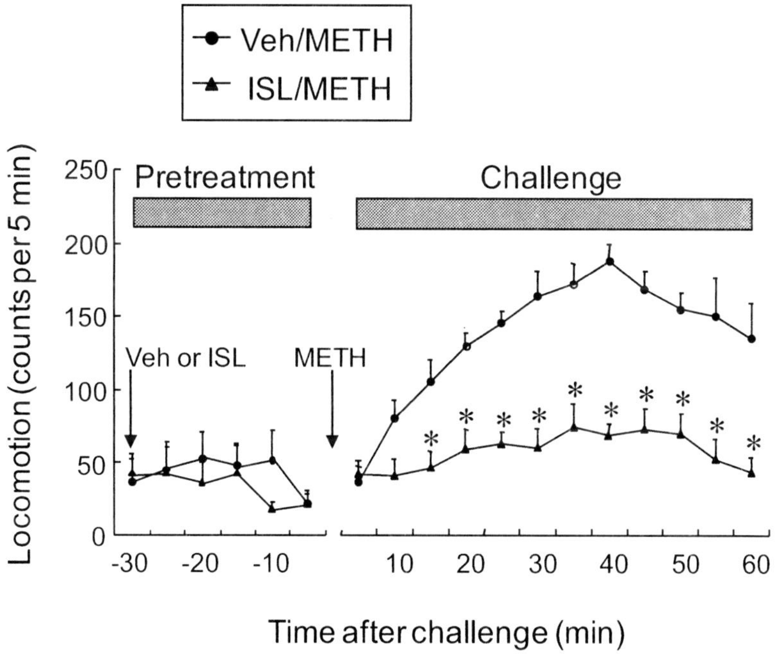

Figure 1. Effect of isoliquiritigenin (ISL; 20 mg/kg, i.p.) on methamphetamine (METH; 1 mg/kg, i.p.)-induced hyperlocomotion in mice (mean ± SEM, $n = 7$ per group). Veh, vehicle for isoliquiritigenin. *$P < 0.05$, compared with Veh/METH-treated group (Bonferroni/Dunn test).

Table 1. Effect of isoliquiritigenin on tissue levels of monoamines and their metabolites in brain regions of mice challenged with methamphetamine

Brain region	Pretreatment	NE	MHPG	5-HT	5-HIAA
Cerebral cortex	Vehicle	0.480 ± 0.044	0.200 ± 0.016	0.647 ± 0.050	0.243 ± 0.022
	ISL	0.487 ± 0.029	0.223 ± 0.022	0.621 ± 0.015	0.226 ± 0.024
Striatum + NAc	Vehicle	0.688 ± 0.058	0.176 ± 0.024	1.003 ± 0.109	0.574 ± 0.042
	ISL	0.675 ± 0.047	0.170 ± 0.011	0.989 ± 0.116	0.547 ± 0.047
Thalamus +	Vehicle	2.129 ± 0.069	0.188 ± 0.011	1.665 ± 0.015	0.644 ± 0.024
hypothalamus	ISL	2.060 ± 0.065	0.187 ± 0.012	1.625 ± 0.058	0.625 ± 0.039
Brain region	Pretreatment	DA	DOPAC	3-MT	HVA
Cerebral cortex	Vehicle	1.273 ± 0.264	0.099 ± 0.016	0.044 ± 0.008	0.152 ± 0.011
	ISL	0.952 ± 0.262	0.069 ± 0.015	0.045 ± 0.014	0.124 ± 0.024
Striatum + NAc	Vehicle	5.839 ± 0.330	0.373 ± 0.021	0.253 ± 0.059	0.515 ± 0.035
	ISL	5.325 ± 0.459	0.376 ± 0.045	0.258 ± 0.040	0.477 ± 0.034
Thalamus +	Vehicle	0.328 ± 0.017	0.128 ± 0.008	N.D.	0.145 ± 0.009
hypothalamus	ISL	0.343 ± 0.035	0.115 ± 0.010	N.D.	0.135 ± 0.011

The brains were dissected 40 min after METH challenge. Values are expressed as nanograms per milligram of wet tissue (mean ± SEM, $n = 6$). DOPAC, 3:4-dihydroxyphenylacetic acid; DA, dopamine; 5-HIAA, 5-hydroxyindolacetic acid; 5-HT, 5-hydroxytryptamine (serotonin); HVA, homovanillic acid; ISL, isoliquiritigenin; METH, methamphetamine; MHPG, 3-methoxy-4-hydroxy-phenylglycol; 3-MT, 3-methoxytyramine; NAc, nucleus accumbens; N.D., not detected; NE, norepinephrine.

A repeated-measures ANOVA (Pretreatment x Time) applied to the data represented in Figure 1 (Time = 0-60 min after challenge) revealed significant main effects of Time ($F(11,144) = 9.100$, $P < 0.0001$) and Pretreatment ($F(1,144) = 67.034$, $P < 0.0001$) and a significant Pretreatment x Time interaction ($F(11,144) = 3.628$, $P < 0.001$). Bonferroni-corrected pairwise comparisons found that ISL pretreatment significantly decreased locomotor activity after METH challenge at the time of 15 min and later ($P < 0.05$).

Effect of ISL on Tissue Levels of Monoamines and their Metabolites in Brain Regions of Mice Challenged with METH

As shown in Figure 1, maximal inhibition by ISL of METH-induced hyperlocomotion was observed 40 min after METH challenge. Therefore, tissue contents of monoamines and their metabolites were determined in the mice 40 min after METH challenge. Mice were treated with ISL or vehicle (n = 6 per group) for 30 min followed by METH challenge. Forty minutes later, the brains were immediately removed and dissected for HPLC analysis. Table 1 shows a summary of the tissue levels of monoamines and their metabolites in the cerebral cortex, the region of striatum and nucleus accumbens, and the region of thalamus and hypothalamus.

One-way ANOVA (Pretreatment) applied to the cerebral cortex showed no significant main effects of Pretreatment for all monoamines and their metabolites ($F(1,10) = 0.016$, $P = 0.9021$, $F(1,10) = 0.692$, $P = 0.4248$, $F(1,10) = 0.235$, $P = 0.6384$, $F(1,10) = 0.271$, $P = 0.6138$, $F(1,10) = 0.742$, $P = 0.4092$, $F(1,10) = 1.849$, $P = 0.2037$, $F(1,10) = 0.003$, $P = 0.9568$, and $F(1,10) = 1.174$, $P = 0.3040$ for NE, MHPG, 5-HT, 5-HIAA, DA, DOPAC, 3-MT, and HVA, respectively). The ANOVA (Pretreatment) applied to the region of striatum and nucleus accumbens showed no significant main effects of Pretreatment for all monoamines and their metabolites ($F(1,10) = 0.034$, $P = 0.8567$, $F(1,10) = 0.054$, $P = 0.8203$, $F(1,10) = 0.008$, $P = 0.9325$, $F(1,10) = 0.176$, $P = 0.6835$, $F(1,10) = 0.825$, $P = 0.3850$, $F(1,10) = 0.003$, $P = 0.9567$, $F(1,10) = 0.006$, $P = 0.9423$, and $F(1,10) = 0.605$, $P = 0.4545$ for NE, MHPG, 5-HT, 5-HIAA, DA, DOPAC, 3-MT, and HVA, respectively). The ANOVA (Pretreatment) applied to the region of thalamus and hypothalamus showed no significant main effects of Pretreatment for all monoamines and their metabolites except 3-MT (which was not detected in either case) ($F(1,10) = 0.531$, $P = 0.4830$, $F(1,10) = 0.004$, $P = 0.9527$, $F(1,10) = 0.436$, $P = 0.5238$, $F(1,10) = 0.165$, $P = 0.6930$, $F(1,10) = 0.143$, $P = 0.7128$, $F(1,10) = 0.932$, P

= 0.3571, and $F(1,10) = 0.488$, $P = 0.5006$ for NE, MHPG, 5-HT, 5-HIAA, DA, DOPAC, and HVA, respectively). Overall, ISL did not affect tissue levels of monoamines and their metabolites in the examined brain regions of the mice challenged with METH.

Effect of ISL on METH-Induced CPP

Figure 2 shows the CPP for METH and the effect of ISL pretreatment on mice. Two-way ANOVA (Pretreatment x Challenge) revealed a significant main effect of Challenge ($F(1,20) = 13.476$, $P < 0.01$), but no significant main effect of Pretreatment ($F(1,20) = 0.005$, $P = 0.9431$) and Pretreatment x Challenge interaction ($F(1,20) = 0.234$, $P = 0.6335$). Bonferroni-corrected pairwise comparisons found that the CPP for METH challenge was significantly increased compared with that observed in the control animals (i.e. saline/saline conditioning group) ($P < 0.05$).

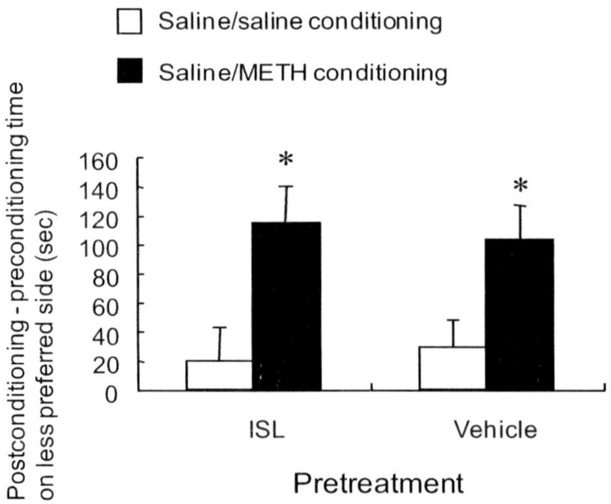

Figure 2. Conditioned place preference (CPP) for methamphetamine (METH) and the effect of isoliquiritigenin (ISL) pretreatment in mice. Place preference was measured as the difference in the time spent in the less preferred compartment associated with saline (open column) or METH (0.5 mg/kg) (closed column) between the post-conditioning and preconditioning sessions (mean ± SEM, $n = 6$ per group). Mice were injected with ISL (20 mg/kg) or vehicle (Veh) 30 min prior to saline or METH conditioning and confined to an assigned compartment for 20 min. *$P < 0.05$, compared with saline/saline conditioning (Bonferroni/Dunn test).

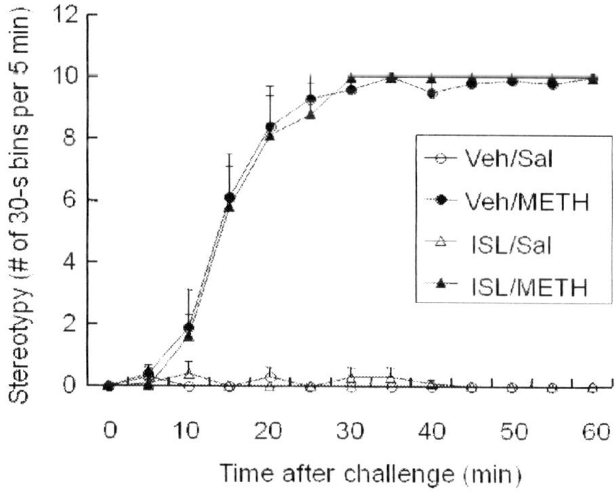

Figure 3. Frequency of stereotypy observed after a single administration of methamphetamine (METH; 10 mg/kg). Values are shown as means ± SEM ($n = 8$ per group). ISL, isoliquiritigenin (20 mg/kg); Sal, saline; Veh, vehicle.

Effect of ISL on METH-Induced Stereotypy and Horizontal Locomotion

Figure 3 shows the time course of the frequency of all stereotypical behavior after METH (or saline vehicle) challenge in mice. There was an increase in the overall frequency of stereotypy in mice after METH challenge, compared with that for saline challenge, beginning at 5 min post-injection, reaching a maximum at 30 min post-injection, and continuing unabated for the duration of the test session. The frequency of stereotypy was unchanged after pretreatment with 20 mg/kg ISL or vehicle for ISL overall. There was no change in the total frequency of METH-induced stereotypy over time as a result of ISL pretreatment. A repeated-measures ANOVA (Pretreatment x Challenge x Time) applied to the data represented in Figure 3 yielded significant main effects of Challenge ($F(1,28) = 1452.102$, $P < 0.0001$) and Time ($F(12,336) = 74.899$, $P < 0.0001$), but no significant main effect of Pretreatment ($F(1,28) = 0.006$, $P = 0.9397$). This analysis also yielded a significant Challenge x Time interaction ($F(12,336) = 77.199$, $P < 0.0001$), but no significant Pretreatment x Challenge, Pretreatment x Time, or Pretreatment x Challenge x Time interaction ($F(1,28) = 0.032$, $P = 0.8599$, $F(12,336) = 0.191$, $P = 0.9988$, and $F(12,336) = 0.116$, $P > 0.9999$, respectively). *Post hoc* pairwise comparisons showed significant differences of time course between the time of 5 min and the time of 10-60 min, between the time of 10 min and the time of 15-60 min, and between the time of 15 min and the time of 20-60 min (Bonferroni/Dunn test, $P < 0.05$).

Four categories of stereotyped behaviors were observed and the frequency of each behavior was measured for 1 h (Figure 4A-D). The total counts of all observed stereotypical behaviors (head-bobbing + circling + sniffing + biting) and persistent locomotion are also shown in Figure 4E and F, respectively. METH challenge increased the frequency of each category of stereotyped behavior (except circling) and persistent locomotion, compared with saline challenge (essentially none of these behaviors was observed after saline injection). Two-way ANOVA (Pretreatment x Challenge) was applied separately for each behavior shown in Figure 4A-D and F. The ANOVA showed significant main effects of Challenge ($F(1,28) = 6.488$, $P < 0.05$, $F(1,28) = 18.000$, $P < 0.001$, $F(1,28) = 1077.323$, $P < 0.0001$, and $F(1,28) = 52.968$, $P < 0.0001$ for head-bobbing, sniffing, biting, and persistent locomotion, respectively, but no significant main effect of Challenge for circling, $F(1,28) = 1.000$, $P = 0.3259$). Furthermore, pretreatment with ISL significantly affected the expression of sniffing, but not head-bobbing, circling, biting, and persistent locomotion. Thus, there was a significant main effect of Pretreatment for sniffing ($F(1,28) = 6.612$, $P < 0.05$), but no significant main effects of Pretreatment for head-bobbing, circling, biting, and persistent locomotion ($F(1,28) = 1.104$, $P = 0.3226$, $F(1,28) = 1.000$, $P = 0.3259$, $F(1,28) = 0.444$, $P = 0.5109$, and $F(1,28) = 0.004$, $P = 0.9496$, respectively). The frequency of METH-induced stereotypical sniffing was significantly enhanced by pretreatment with ISL. Thus, the ANOVA also indicated a significant Pretreatment x Challenge interaction for sniffing ($F(1,28) = 4.231$, $P < 0.05$), but no significant Pretreatment x Challenge interactions for head-bobbing, circling, biting, and persistent locomotion ($F(1,28) = 1.104$, $P = 0.3226$, $F(1,28) = 1.000$, $P = 0.3259$, $F(1,28) = 0.509$, $P = 0.4814$, and $F(1,28) = 0.004$, $P = 0.9496$, respectively). Regarding the METH challenge, *post hoc* comparisons indicated significant differences in the frequencies of the stereotypical behavior components except circling between the METH-treated and the saline-treated mice (Bonferroni/Dunn test, $P < 0.05$). Despite these differences in the frequency of individual stereotypical behaviors, the total incidence of stereotypy was unaffected. A separate two-way ANOVA applied to the total frequency of stereotypic behavior represented in Figure 4E indicated a significant main effect of Challenge ($F(1,28) = 1452.102$, $P < 0.0001$), but no significant main effect of Pretreatment ($F(1,28) = 0.006$, $P = 0.9397$). The ANOVA also showed no significant Pretreatment x Challenge interaction ($F(1,28) = 0.032$, $P = 0.8599$) for the total frequency of four stereotypical behaviors. Regarding the METH challenge, *post hoc* comparisons indicated a significant difference of frequencies of total stereotyped behavior between the METH-treated and the saline-treated mice (Bonferroni/Dunn test, $P < 0.05$).

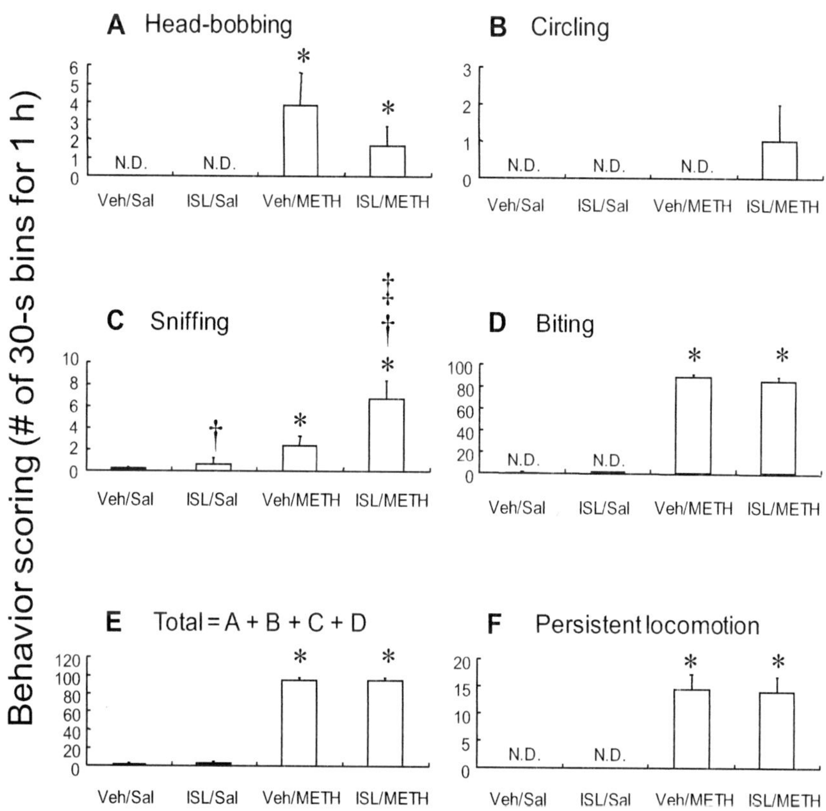

Figure 4. Stereotyped behavior in response to saline (Sal) or methamphetamine (METH) in mice pretreated with 20 mg/kg isoliquiritigenin (ISL) or vehicle. Behavior was scored in 30-s bins, and total numbers for 1 h are shown. A, Head-bobbing; B, circling; C, sniffing; D, nail and/or wood-chip biting; E, total number of stereotypic scores ("Total") includes the numbers of head-bobbing, circling, sniffing, and nail and/or wood-chip biting. Values are shown as means ± SEM ($n = 8$ per group). $^*P < 0.05$, compared with saline challenge (Bonferroni/Dunn test). $^\dagger P < 0.05$, compared with vehicle pretreatment (Bonferroni/Dunn test). ISL pretreatment significantly enhanced METH-induced stereotypical sniffing compared with that induced by METH after vehicle ($^\ddagger P < 0.05$, compared with Veh/METH). N.D., not detected.

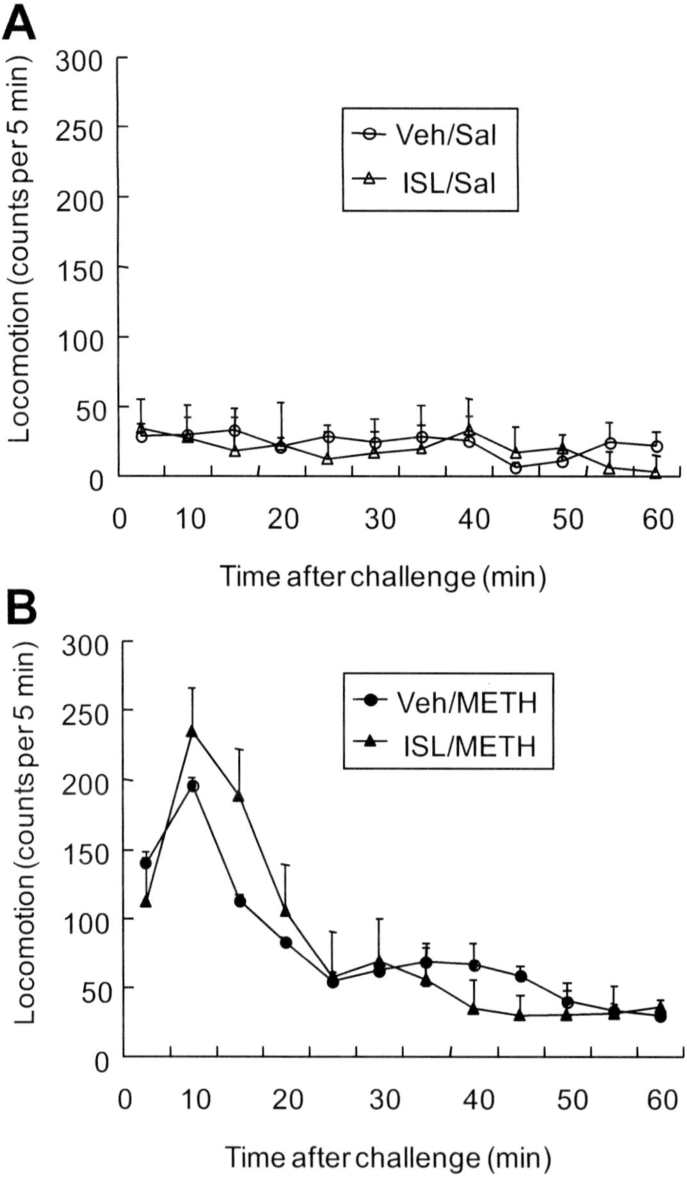

Figure 5. Locomotor activity after a single administration of saline (A) or methamphetamine (METH; 10 mg/kg) (B) in mice pretreated with 20 mg/kg isoliquiritigenin (ISL) or vehicle (Veh). Values are shown as means ± SEM (n = 8 per group). Sal, saline.

METH treatment increased locomotion compared with saline treatment, but ISL did not substantially affect locomotion in either case. Locomotor activity was analyzed by separate repeated-measures ANOVA (Pretreatment x Time) applied to the saline-treated (Figure 5A) and METH-treated (Figure 5B) subjects. There was a significant main effect of Time for METH-treated mice ($F(11,168) = 12.817$, $P < 0.0001$), but no significant main effect of Time for saline-treated mice ($F(11,168) = 1.071$, $P = 0.3881$). There were no significant main effects of Pretreatment for saline-treated ($F(1,14) = 0.566$, $P = 0.4645$) and METH-treated ($F(1,14) = 0.049$, $P = 0.8288$) mice. The Pretreatment x Challenge interaction was also not significant ($F(11,168) = 0.774$, $P = 0.6652$), nor was it for METH-treated ($F(11,168) = 0.951$, $P = 0.4935$). Overall, ISL did not affect locomotor activity alone or METH-induced hyperactivity.

DISCUSSION

In the present study, we demonstrated that pretreatment of mice with ISL significantly inhibited METH-induced hyperlocomotion (Figure 1). The inhibitory effect of ISL on behavior was specific for METH-induced hyperlocomotion, since (1) METH-induced CPP or total incidence of stereotypy was unaffected by ISL pretreatment (Figs. 2 and 3), (2) ISL itself had no effect on spontaneous locomotion during the pretreatment period (Figure 1), and (3) pretreatment with ISL had no effect on locomotor activity after saline challenge (Figure 5A).

The difference of locomotor activities between ISL-pretreated mice and those pretreated with vehicle peaked 40 min after METH injection (Figure 1). Thus, tissue levels of monoamines and their metabolites were measured in the brain regions of mice pretreated with ISL (or vehicle) 40 min after the METH injection, in order to investigate a possible association of ISL pretreatment with alterations of monoamines and their metabolites. As shown in Table 1, there were no significant alterations in tissue levels of monoamines and their metabolites in the cerebral cortex, the region of the striatum and the NAc, and the region of the thalamus and hypothalamus between mice pretreated with ISL and vehicle. Therefore, the results suggest that ISL inhibits METH-induced hyperlocomotion by a mechanism independent of monoamine metabolism.

Pretreatment of rats with ISL inhibits cocaine-induced extracellular DA release in the NAc (Jang et al., 2008). This ISL action may account for the inhibitory effect of ISL on cocaine-induced hyperlocomotion (Jeon et al., 2008). A single administration of METH (1 mg/kg, i.p.) to mice increases extracellular DA release in the NAc (Shimosato et al., 2003) and increases and decreases tissue contents of DA and DOPAC, respectively, in the region of striatum and NAc (Kitanaka et al., 2003, 2005). Provided that ISL pretreatment inhibits METH-induced extracellular DA release in the NAc, the tissue level of DA and that of DOPAC decreases and increases, respectively, in the striatum and NAc of mice pretreated with ISL compared with those pretreated with vehicle. This is not the case in the present study (Table 1), suggesting that the inhibitory effect of ISL on METH-induced hyperlocomotion is not mediated primarily by ISL suppression of extracellular DA release in the NAc. Again, it is not likely that ISL inhibits METH-induced extracellular DA release in the NAc because CPP or stereotypical behavior induced by METH was unaffected by ISL pretreatment (Figs. 2 and 3).

ISL pretreatment significantly increased sniffing behavior in mice challenged with saline, and enhanced METH-induced stereotypical sniffing compared with that of vehicle-pretreated mice (Figure 4C). This suggests that ISL may be anxiogenic because sniffing behavior is associated with anxiety (Blanchard et al., 2000). Alternatively, METH-induced stereotypical sniffing is significantly enhanced by pretreatment with histamine *N*-methyltransferase inhibitors (metoprine and SKF 91488), histamine H_3 receptor antagonists (thioperamide and clobenpropit), or sigma$_1$ receptor antagonists (BMY 14802 and BD 1047) (Kitanaka et al., 2007, 2009, 2010). In line with these observations, it is possible that ISL enhances hypothalamic levels of histamine, or it might interact with sigma$_1$ receptor sites with a possible antagonistic property, resulting in the enhancement of METH-induced stereotypical sniffing by ISL pretreatment. This speculation needs to be clarified in further studies.

Taking these findings together, pretreatment with ISL selectively inhibited METH-induced hyperlocomotion in mice. The mechanism is currently uncertain, but unlike cocaine studies (Jang et al., 2008; Jeon et al., 2008), the inhibitory ISL action on METH-induced hyperlocomotion is not likely to be mediated by suppression of DAnergic neurotransmission in the NAc.

ACKNOWLEDGMENT

The authors are grateful to Ms. A. Yoshioka of the Department of Pharmacology, Hyogo College of Medicine, for preparing the animal study proposal. This research was supported, in part, by a Grant-in-Aid for Young Scientists (B) from the Ministry of Education, Culture, Sports, Science, and Technology of Japan (No. 21790254 to N.K.) and by a Grant-in-Aid for Researchers from the Hyogo College of Medicine (2009-2010 to J.K.).

REFERENCES

Blanchard RJ, Hebert M, Dulloog L, Markham C, Figueira R, Nishimura O, Newsham K, Kaawaloa JN, Blanchard DC (2000) Cocaine-induced sniffing stereotypy changes in response to threat. *Pharmacol Biochem Behav* 66:249-256.

Chin YW, Jung HA, Liu Y, Su BN, Castoro JA, Keller WJ, Pereira MA, Kinghorn AD (2007) Anti-oxidant constituents of the roots and stolons of licorice (*Glycyrrhiza glabra*). *J Agric Food Chem 55*:4691-4697.

Di Chiara G, Imperato A (1988) Drugs abused by humans preferentially increase synaptic DA concentrations in the mesolimbic system of freely moving rats. *Proc Natl Acad Sci USA* 85:5274-5278.

Jang EY, Choe ES, Hwang M, Kim SC, Lee JR, Kim SG, Jeon J-P, Buono RJ, Yang CH (2008) Isoliquiritigenin suppresses cocaine-induced extracellular dopamine release in rat brain through $GABA_B$ receptor. *Eur J Pharmacol* 587:124-128.

Jeon JP, Buono RJ, Han BG, Jang EY, Kim SC, Yang CH, Hwang M (2008) Proteomic and behavioral analysis of response to Isoliquilitigenin in brains of acute cocaine treated rats. *J Proteome Res* 7:5094-5102.

Kantak KM (2003) Vaccines against drugs of abuse: a viable treatment option? *Drugs* 63:341-352.

Kitanaka J, Kitanaka N, Tatsuta T, Morita Y, Takemura M (2007) Blockade of brain histamine metabolism alters methamphetamine-induced expression patteren of stereotypy in mice via histamine H_1 receptors. *Neuroscience* 147:765-777.

Kitanaka J, Kitanaka N, Tatsuta T, Hall FS, Uhl GR, Tanaka K, Nishiyama N, Morita Y, Takemura M (2009) $Sigma_1$ receptor antagonists determine the behavioral pattern of the methamphetamine-induced stereotypy in mice. *Psychopharmacology (Berl)* 203:781-792.

Kitanaka J, Kitanaka N, Tatsuta T, Miyoshi A, Koumoto A, Tanaka K, Nishiyama N, Morita Y, Takemura M (2010) Pretreatment with L-histidine produces a shift from methamphetamine-induced stereotypical biting to persistent locomotion in mice. *Pharmacol Biochem Behav* 94:464-470.

Kitanaka N, Kitanaka J, Takemura M (2003) Behavioral sensitization and alteration in monoamine metabolism in mice after single versus repeated methamphetamine administration. *Eur J Pharmacol* 474:63-70.

Kitanaka N, Kitanaka J, Takemura M (2005) Inhibition of methamphetamine-induced hyperlocomotion in mice by clorgyline, a monoamine oxidase-A inhibitor, through alteration of the 5-hydroxytryptamine turnover in the striatum. *Neuroscience* 130:295-308.

Kitanaka N, Kitanaka J, Tatsuta T, Watabe K, Morita Y, Takemura M (2006) Methamphetamine reward in mice as assessed by conditioned place preference test with Supermex® sensors: effect of subchronic clorgyline pretreatment. *Neurochem Res* 31:805-813.

Mori T, Ito S, Kita T, Sawaguchi T (2004) Effects of dopamine- and serotonin-related compounds on methamphetamine-induced self-injurious behavior in mice. *J Pharmacol Sci* 96:459-464.

National Institute on Drug Abuse (2004) NIDA InfoFacts: methamphetamine. Accessed 17 Dec 2010. URL: http://www.drugabuse.gov/infofacts/methamphetamine.html

Seiden LS, Sabol KE, Ricaurte GA (1993) Amphetamine: effects on catecholamine systems and behavior. *Annu Rev Pharmacol Toxicol* 32:639-677.

Shimosato K, Nagao N, Watanabe S, Kitayama S (2003) Suppressive effects of trihexyphenidyl on methamphetamine-induced dopamine release as measured by in vivo microdialysis. *Synapse* 49:47-54.

Srisurapanont M, Jarusuraisin N, Kittirattanapaiboon P (2001) Treatment for amphetamine dependence and abuse. *Cochrane Database Syst Rev* 4:CD003022.

Sulzer D, Sonders MS, Poulsen NW, Galli A (2005) Mechanisms of neurotransmitter release by amphetamines: a review. *Prog Neurobiol* 75:406-433.

Tada M, Shirakawa K, Matsuoka N, Mutoh S (2004) Combined treatment of quetiapine with haloperidol in animal models of antipsychotic effect and extrapyramidal side effects: comparison with risperidone and chlorpromazine. *Psychopharmacology* (Berl) 176:94-100.

Ujike H, Sato M (2004) Clinical features of sensitization to methamphetamine observed in patients with methamphetamine dependence and psychosis. *Ann NY Acad Sci* 1025:279-287.

Yamamoto S, Aizu E, Jiang H, Nakadate T, Kiyoton I, Wang JC, Kato R (1991) The potent anti-tumor-promoting agent isoliquiritigenin. *Carcinogenesis* 12:317-323.

In: Methamphetamines
Editors: J. Ornoy and X. He

ISBN: 978-1-62100-244-4

Chapter 6

DIFFERENCES AMONG METHAMPHETAMINE AND COCAINE DEPENDENT PREGNANT AND PARENTING WOMEN ENROLLED IN AN OUTPATIENT TREATMENT PROGRAM

***Sabrina D. Diaz*[1], *Jennifer H. Kuo*[1], *Toni Wallace*[2], *Carol D. Berkowitz*[1], *M. Lynn Yonekura*[2], and *Lynne M. Smith*[1,*]**

[1]Department of Pediatrics, Harbor-UCLA Medical Center and David Geffen School of Medicine at UCLA, Los Angeles, CA, US
[2]Department of Obstetrics, Harbor-UCLA Medical Center, Torrance, CA, US

ABSTRACT

Background: Gender differences in substance abusing populations have been examined, with some drug treatment strategies found to be more successful for women than for men. Although the female adult cocaine-using population has been well characterized, less is known about the characteristics of the female adult methamphetamine (MA) user.

* Correspondence to: Lynne M. Smith, M.D. Professor of Pediatrics. David Geffen School of Medicine, Harbor-UCLA Medical Center, 1124 West Carson Street, Box 446, Torrance, CA 90502; Telephone (310) 222-1968. Fax: (310) 222-3887; E-mail: smith@labiomed.org.

Objective: To determine the similarities and differences between MA- and cocaine-dependent pregnant and parenting women.

Design: We conducted a retrospective review of women enrolled in the Stork Club, an outpatient drug treatment program for pregnant and parenting women (n=202). Demographics, drug use history, education/ employment status prior to treatment, and treatment discharge information were obtained from medical chart reviews using the Los Angeles County Participant Registration Reporting System. Psychiatric symptomatology was assessed using the Psychosocial Assessment Questionnaire. Continuous variables were analyzed using two-tailed t-tests and categorical variables with chi-square tests. Significance was accepted at $P<0.05$.

Results: The cocaine-using women (n=100) were more likely to be homeless (P=0.003), recipients of public assistance (P= 0.03), engage in criminal activity during treatment (P=0.0001), consume alcohol (P=0.02) and drop out of treatment after unsatisfactory progress (P=0.03). In contrast, the MA-using women (n=102) were more likely to successfully complete the treatment program (P=0.02) and own a vehicle (P=0.03); however they were more likely to have contact with intravenous drug users (P=0.01), use a needle within the past year (P=0.01), and use drugs more than once per day at discharge (P=0.01) than the cocaine-using women. Both substance abusing groups had a high incidence of mood disorders. There were no differences in the incidence or types of psychiatric symptomatology between the groups.

Discussion: These findings suggest there are significant differences between MA- and cocaine-using women, with MA-using women facing fewer social barriers. However MA-using women are potentially higher risk for Hepatitis C and HIV due to an increased likelihood of exposure to intravenous drug use. Implications of our findings include the benefits of tailoring treatment and prevention programs to specific substances of abuse.

INTRODUCTION

Substance abuse continues to be a significant problem in the United States, as demonstrated by the 2009 Substance Abuse and Mental Health Services Administration report of 21.8 million current illicit drug users, 1.4 million of whom were women [1]. The Treatment Episode Data Set, a national database obtained from admissions to substance abuse treatment centers, reported 13% of admissions are due to cocaine use (40% females) and 8% are due to methamphetamine (MA) use (46% females) [2]. Although cocaine and MA are both psychostimulants, researchers have found stark differences in user characteristics and consequences of use. MA has a much longer half life than cocaine, 8-14 hours compared to 20-30 minutes, possibly impacting some of the differences. The literature on primarily males reports cocaine users are more likely to be African-American [3], married [3], to use less frequently but in higher quantity [3], and consume more alcohol [3,4], whereas MA users are more likely to be female [3], gay/bisexual, HIV-positive, use needles for drug administration, have contact with other intravenous drug users [4], have medical and psychiatric consequences [3,4], and problems with manipulating information, perseveration and set shifting [5].

Gender-specific substance abuse research has only recently emerged. Males generally have higher usage rates for most illicit drugs, including cocaine; however males and females have reported similar rates of MA use [1]. Given that gender-specific substance abuse treatment has been found to be more effective for females [6,7], it is necessary to better characterize the female substance abuser to design effective treatment strategies. Due to the widespread use of cocaine in the United States since the 1980s, both the male and female cocaine-using population has been well characterized. Researchers have found gender-based differences including increased incidence of depressive symptoms and psychiatric disorders in female cocaine users [8,9], female cocaine users being more likely to be unemployed, hold lower paying jobs [10,8,9], progressing to drug dependence more rapidly than males [10], and less likely to be involved in criminal activities [10]. These findings have helped drug treatment programs tailor therapy to address the specific needs of the female cocaine-using population.

Because the emergence of MA use is more recent, less is known about the characteristics of the female MA-using population. A prospective longitudinal study in California found in comparison to male MA users, female MA users are more likely to be younger, unemployed, on public assistance, experience serious depression and thoughts of suicide, prescribed medication for a psychological problem, and less likely to be on parole [11,12]. Female MA users are also more likely to use on consecutive days, use MA for energy and weight loss, and less likely to have work problems, high blood pressure or use hallucinogens, crack, inhalants, PCP, heroin and downers [13]. Researchers have also found high rates of social isolation, chaotic home life, family conflict, and interpersonal difficulties among female MA users [14]. Female MA users are more likely to attempt suicide, exhibit violent behavior problems, and have higher inventory scores on all nine dimensions of the Brief Symptom Inventory (anxiety, depression, hostility, interpersonal sensitivity, obsessive-compulsive, paranoid ideation, phobic anxiety, psychoticism and somatization) compared to male MA users [15]; however in a study of women who used MA during pregnancy, no association was found with MA use and psychological distress [16].

We chose to study the similarities and differences between MA- and cocaine-using women enrolled in the Stork Club, an outpatient drug treatment program, to investigate whether gender-specific substance abuse treatment should be further altered depending on the specific drug being abused. The Stork Club provides the same treatment strategies for MA- and cocaine-using clients allowing comparison between the two groups. Based on the differences in male MA- and cocaine-using populations, we hypothesized that we would find differences in demographic and drug use patterns among women that would have potential treatment implications.

Subjects and Methods

The study was approved by the Institutional Review Board prior to initiating work on this project. We retrospectively reviewed medical records of all women with a primary diagnosis of MA or cocaine dependence enrolled in the Stork Club at Harbor-UCLA Medical Center between 1993 and 2000. A total of 202 women (n=102 MA) were reviewed. The Stork Club is a state-funded, intensive day treatment program serving chemically dependent pregnant and parenting women and their infants and toddlers in the South Bay region of Los Angeles, California. Clients are referred from a number of sources; the majority of the women in the program are referred by the Los Angeles County Department of Children's and Family Services; however a few of the clients are self-referred. The incidence of MA users entering the drug treatment program increased significantly during the time period reviewed. In 1993, the percentage of MA- and cocaine-using enrolled in the drug treatment program women was 27 and 56%, respectively. By the year 2000, the percentage of MA users had increased to 43% of the enrollment and cocaine-dependence had decreased to 29% of enrollees. The number of women enrolled at the Stork Club was consistent throughout the study period.

Services are provided to each client six hours a day, five days per week for one year. Scheduled activities (and the number of sessions) per week are as follows: individual counseling (1), group counseling (3), group education (9), employment counseling (1), 12-step meeting (1), Mommy and Me circle time (5), and relaxation training (1). All sessions are at least an hour with the exception of the Mommy and Me circle time that meets for 30-minutes in the mornings before treatment. The clients also undergo observed random weekly drug testing while in the program. Homeless clients and their children are placed in local sober living homes. Transportation assistance is also available in the form of bus tokens.

For 6-months following successful completion of drug/alcohol treatment, graduates participate in aftercare services that consist of a weekly group counseling session and two 12-step sessions per month. The Stork Club also provides referrals to the CalWORKS GAIN employment services program. Clients also receive case management services and may receive group or individual therapy and in-home parenting sessions as needed.

All clients entering the program are interviewed for an intake assessment by staff trained to be non-judgmental and to provide a supportive environment. Staff members have masters or bachelors level degrees with certification in drug and alcohol counseling. Data obtained from standard countywide forms include demographics, drug use history, education/employment status, medical, family, and psychiatric information. Psychiatric symptomatology was assessed by self-report using the Psychosocial Assessment Questionnaire. Clients judged to have significant symptoms were referred to the Harbor-UCLA Medical Center Psychiatric Department for further evaluation.

At the time of discharge from the program, staff members obtained information via self-report regarding the success of treatment, drug history from the past 30 days, employment status, probable criminal activity during treatment, updated medical history, living situation and sexual activity. Success of treatment was broken into the following categories: completed treatment, left treatment with satisfactory progress, left treatment with unsatisfactory progress, and referred or transferred. Successful completion of the program was awarded to clients who attended all required education classes, received a 12-week parenting certificate, and had negative random toxicology screens. Criminal activity was determined by self report of the subject, or from family members and significant others if the subject dropped out.

Statistical Analysis

Demographics, substance use, psychiatric symptomatology and discharge characteristics were examined by primary drug use at time of admission. Means and standard deviations are used for continuous measures. Categorical variables are expressed as observed counts and percentages. Significant levels for differences in drug used were derived from two-tailed Student's t-test and χ^2 tests, as determined by variable type. Significance was accepted for P values <0.05.

RESULTS

Table 1 compares the demographic information of the MA- (n=102) and cocaine-using (n=100) women at time of admission to the program.

Table 1. Demographic characteristics by primary substance abuse at admission

	Number (%) / Mean (SD)		P-Value
	Methamphe-tamine (n=102)	Cocaine (n=100)	
Age	27.7±5.3	29.9±4.6	ns
Ethnicity			
Caucasian	78.4 (79)	20.0 (20)	**0.0001**
African American	0.0 (0)	60.0 (60)	**0.0001**
Hispanic	17.6 (18)	14.0 (14)	ns
Asian/Pacific Islander	2.0 (2)	2.0 (2)	ns
Other	2.0 (2)	4.0 (4)	ns
Homeless	9.8 (10)	26.0 (26)	**0.003**
Married	11.8 (12)	15.0 (15)	ns
Education (years)	11.3±1.4	12.0±1.7	ns
Assistance			
AFDC	25.5 (26)	41.0 (41)	**0.03**
Public insurance	34.3 (35)	47.0 (47)	ns
Own vehicle	21.6 (22)	10.0 (10)	**0.03**
Employment			
Employed	1.0 (1)	2.0 (2)	ns
Seeking employment	7.8 (8)	4.0 (4)	ns
Not seeking employment	84.3 (85)	91.0 (91)	ns
Job training	5.9 (6)	3.0 (3)	ns

There were significant differences in ethnicity between the women with the percent of African Americans in the MA and cocaine-using groups 0 vs.

60%, respectively. In contrast, almost 80% of MA users were Caucasian; however, the percent of Hispanic and Asian/Pacific Islander users was comparable in each group. MA-using women were more likely to own a vehicle (p=0.03) and cocaine-using women were more likely to be homeless (p=0.003) and receive government assistance from Aid to Families with Dependent Children/Temporary Assistance to Needy Families (p=0.03). No differences were found regarding age, marital status, level of education, receiving public insurance, and employment status between the groups upon entry into the program.

Substance use characteristics are shown in Table 2.

Table 2. Substance use characteristics at admission

	Number (%)		P-Value
	Methamphetamine	Cocaine	
Alcohol use	39.2 (40)	56.0 (56)	**0.02**
Sedative use	2.0 (2)	3.0 (3)	ns
Frequency of MA or Cocaine Use			
None in past month	22.6 (23)	25.0 (25)	ns
Less than once per week	16.7 (17)	5.0 (5)	**0.01**
Once per week	3.9 (4)	10.0 (10)	ns
Several times per week	24.5 (25)	24.0 (24)	ns
Once per day	5.9 (6)	3.0 (3)	ns
More than once per day	26.5 (27)	33.0 (33)	ns
Route of Administration			
Oral	2.0 (2)	2.0 (2)	ns
Smoking	49.0 (49)	94.0 (94)	**0.0001**
Inhalation	38.2 (39)	6.0 (6)	**0.0001**
Needle use in the past year	14.7 (15)	3.0 (3)	**0.01**
Sexual contact with IV drug user	26.5 (27)	12.0 (12)	**0.01**

The cocaine-using women were more likely to consume alcohol at admission than the MA-using women (p=0.02). MA-using women were more likely to consume MA less than once per week (p=0.01), although there are no differences between groups for abstinence or higher frequency of illicit drug use. Cocaine users were more likely to smoke their cocaine, whereas MA users were more likely to use inhalation as the primary route of drug administration (p=0.0001); MA users were more likely to use needles and to have had sexual contact with an intravenous drug user (p=0.01). Table 3 shows the prevalence of psychiatric symptomatology.

Table 3. Psychiatric symptomatology

	Number (%)		P-Value
	Methamphetamine	Cocaine	
Mood Disorder	22.5 (23)	17.0 (17)	ns
Anxiety Disorder	5.9 (6)	8.0 (8)	ns
Thought Disorder	0.0 (0)	6.0 (6)	ns
Personality Disorder	11.8 (12)	9.0 (9)	ns
Eating Disorder	0.0 (0)	1.0 (1)	ns
Attention Deficit Disorder	1.0 (1)	0.0 (0)	ns

Table 4. Characteristics and drug use frequency at discharge from the program

	Number (%)		P-Value
	Methamphe-tamine (n=102)	Cocaine (n=100)	
Discharge status			
Completed Treatment	40.2 (41)	25.0 (25)	**0.02**
Left, satisfactory condition	8.8 (9)	8.0 (8)	ns
Left, unsatisfactory condition	45.1 (42)	52.0 (52)	**0.03**
Referred/transferred	0.0 (0)	7.0 (7)	ns
Criminal activity during treatment			
Probable	3.9 (4)	37.0 (37)	**0.0001**
None	45.1 (42)	16.0 (16)	**0.0001**
Unknown	51.0 (51)	47.0 (47)	ns
Employment status at discharge			
Employed	4.9 (5)	6.0 (6)	ns
Unemployed	76.5 (77)	82.0 (82)	ns
Job training	8.8 (9)	0.0 (0)	**0.003**
Frequency of use at discharge			
No use in prior month	57.8 (58)	52.0 (52)	ns
Less than once per week	7.8 (8)	5.0 (5)	ns
Several times per week	2.0 (2)	5.0 (5)	ns
More than once per day	20.0 (20)	6.0 (6)	**0.01**
Needle use for IVDU	2.9 (3)	0.0 (0)	ns

Although several disorders were present in the groups, there were no significant differences in regards to prevalence based on self-report.

MA users were more likely than cocaine users to have successfully completed the treatment program (41 vs. 25% respectively, P=0.02) and cocaine users were more likely to leave the treatment program with unsatisfactory progress (52 vs. 42% respectively, P=0.03) (Table 4).

Unsatisfactory progress is defined as not attending classes, having positive urine toxicology screens, or breaking treatment contracts. Unsatisfactory progress is often followed by either a referral to a different treatment program or withdrawal from the Stork Club. The cocaine-using women showed more probable criminal activity during the course of treatment (P=0.0001). There were no differences in employment status at the time of discharge from the program although a small but significant number of MA-exposed women were in a job-training program. Additionally there were no differences in frequency of drug use or needle use at the time of discharge, with the exception of frequent daily use by MA-exposed women (P=0.01).

CONCLUSION

This study examines the characteristics of MA- and cocaine-using pregnant and parenting women. Previous studies comparing primarily male MA and cocaine users found differences in ethnicity and risk-taking behaviors such as IV drug use between the two groups [3,4]. Our findings are consistent with these observations. We found women who use cocaine were more likely to be African-American; whereas MA-using women were more likely to be Caucasian. MA users were also more likely to administer drugs intravenously and to have had contact with other intravenous drug users. In contrast to previous observations involving primarily males, we found MA users were more likely than cocaine users to successfully complete the drug treatment program [17,4,3].

Our findings of increased needle use and contact with intravenous drug users in the MA-users relative to cocaine users at time of admission are consistent with work by Copeland and colleagues in male MA users [4]. Needle use and contact with intravenous drug users are major risk factors for contracting HIV and hepatitis C [18]. Over one million people in the United States are living with HIV and women account for 27% of annual new HIV infections [19]. Additionally, hepatitis C is currently the leading cause for liver transplantation in the United States [20]. Intravenous drug abuse not only endangers the health of these women, but also poses significant risks to the fetus. Although current antiretroviral therapy has minimized the risk of HIV transmission to the fetus, there is no known therapy to prevent placental transmission of hepatitis C. Given the high intravenous exposure rate in MA women and the fact that HIV and hepatitis C infections may produce few symptoms initially, screening of HIV and hepatitis C should be routine in this high risk population. The American Association for the Study of Liver Diseases recommends that any person who has ever injected illegal drugs, once or continuously, should have routine HCV testing [21]. Thus, HCV and HIV testing is recommended to all patients seeking drug treatment, especially for IV use.

We found no differences in psychiatric symptomatology between MA- and cocaine-using pregnant and parenting women. These findings are in contrast to previous observations that MA-using individuals in treatment have higher rates of psychiatric disorders relative to cocaine users [4,3], however these studies did not examine gender differences. Copeland and colleagues found approximately half of MA users had psychiatric symptoms whereas psychiatric symptoms were identified in only 28% of the cocaine-using group. The disparity between our findings and those previously published may be attributed to the high incidence of males in the previous reports and that substance abusing females are more likely to have a psychiatric disorder than males [22]. However our findings of 40% overall concurrent psychiatric diagnoses in both groups is consistent with previous data showing that 30-60% of cocaine-using patients present with psychiatric disorders [23]. This is possibly attributed to evidence that shows both female MA- and cocaine-using patients are more likely to have a history of sexual and/or physical abuse than male users [24,25,26]. While our study did not gather information regarding the prevalence of sexual and physical abuse, these findings highlight the need for more extensive intake interviews that cover a wider range of questions in order to tailor the treatment programs around the patient.

One study of both male and female MA and cocaine users found only 18% successfully completed a six-month treatment program, but there was no retention difference between the MA and cocaine users [4]. In contrast, approximately one-third of the subjects in our study completed the one-year treatment program. A possible explanation for these differences in success rate may be secondary to our study being limited to pregnant and parenting women. Many of the women require satisfactory completion of their treatment or risk separation from their children by the legal system. A majority of both MA- and cocaine-using women in the treatment program were referred by the

Department of Children and Family Services as contract cases where the mothers sign an agreement stating that if treatment is completed successfully, they will be able to keep their child or have their child returned to them from the foster care system. Hence, our findings of success may be secondary to external forces serving to motivate the population by defining the consequences of not completing the program.

Our findings demonstrate MA-using women were more likely to successfully complete the treatment program than cocaine-using women. The reasons for the apparent enhanced success in MA women are unclear. We found the MA-using women reported less alcohol use and had a lower incidence of homelessness than cocaine-using women. Future studies will need to address whether cocaine users were homeless before they started heavy cocaine use or the homelessness was a result of the drug use. These factors may indicate that the cocaine users in this study had more barriers to completing the treatment program than the MA-using women. In addition, MA using women were more likely to have their own vehicles, making it easier to attend treatment sessions relative to the cocaine using women. However many other, as yet undefined, factors may account for these differences.

Although MA-using women had a higher successful completion rate than CA-using women, MA-using women also demonstrated a higher relapse rate. This may be a result of MA's prolonged impact on the brain dopamine transporters as documented by PET scan [27]. It takes approximately 2 years of complete abstinence for the brain to recover and during that period the client is at high risk for relapse. More recently, investigators have used fMRI activation patterns in the right insular, right posterior cingulate, and right middle temporal gyrus obtained early in recovery to predict relapse susceptibility [28]. MA-dependent subjects who relapsed during follow-up showed less activation in dorsolateral prefrontal, parietal, and temporal cortex, as well as the insula, a network of structures critical for decision making.

Additionally, although there were no differences in employment status between groups at the time of admission, and the majority of all the women were unemployed at time of discharge from the program, significantly more MA users were enrolled in job training upon discharge. This may be related to more MA users owning a vehicle and thus experiencing fewer social barriers [29]. Similarly the lack of criminal activity during treatment by MA users may impact the increase in job training.

There are several limitations to the current investigation so our results should be interpreted with caution. This study utilized a retrospective design, which did not allow for incorporating additional potential variables into the intake questionnaires, such as physical and sexual abuse. The findings are based upon self-report and focus on a specific drug abusing population involved in rehabilitation, not the population at large. Additionally it is unknown whether the intravenous MA use consisted solely of MA or included speedballs, mixtures of MA with heroin. Further longitudinal follow-up is also lacking.

In summary, this retrospective chart review found differences in demographics, substance use characteristics, and rates of treatment completion among pregnant and parenting MA- and cocaine-using women in a drug rehabilitation program. These findings should be incorporated in treatment designs, such that programs are tailored not only toward gender specific treatment, but substance specific treatment as well. Well-designed prospective studies with long-term follow-up are required to better understand the needs of pregnant and parenting drug dependent women and further improve treatment.

Acknowledgment

The authors would like to thank Lorrie Horst, Debra McGrady, and Jillianne Paladino of the Options for Recovery Center at Harbor UCLA Medical Center.

References

[1] Substance Abuse and Mental Health Services Administration 2010. *Results from the 2009 National Survey on Drug Use and Health: Volume I. Summary of National Findings* (NSDUH Series H-38A, HHS Publication No. SMA 10-4856Findings).

[2] *Substance Abuse and Mental Health Services Administration, Office of Applied Studies 2009. Treatment Episode Data Set (TEDS) Highlights* - 2007 National Admissions to Substance Abuse Treatment Services. OAS Series #S-45, Publication No. (SMA) 09-4360.

[3] Rawson, R., Huber, A., Brethen, P., Obert, J., Gulati, V., Shoptaw, S., and Ling, W. Methamphetamine and cocaine users: differences in characteristics and treatment retention. *J Psychoactive Drugs* 2000; 32: 233-238.

[4] Copeland, A. L. and Sorensen, J. L. Differences between methamphetamine users and cocaine users in treatment. *Drug Alcohol Depend* 3-1-2001; 62: 91-95.

[5] Simon, S. L., Domier, C. P., Sim, T., Richardson, K., Rawson, R. A., and Ling, W. Cognitive performance of current methamphetamine and cocaine abusers. *J Addict Dis* 2002; 21: 61-74.

[6] Fattore, L., Altea, S., and Fratta, W. Sex differences in drug addiction: a review of animal and human studies. *Womens Health* (Lond Engl) 2008; 4: 51-65.

[7] Ashley, O. S., Marsden, M. E., and Brady, T. M. Effectiveness of substance abuse treatment programming for women: a review. *Am J Drug Alcohol Abuse* 2003; 29: 19-53.

[8] Griffin, M. L., Weiss, R. D., Mirin, S. M., and Lange, U. A comparison of male and female cocaine abusers. *Arch Gen Psychiatry* 1989; 46: 122-126.

[9] Denier, C. A., Thevos, A. K., Latham, P. K., and Randall, C. L. Psychosocial and psychopathology differences in hospitalized male and female cocaine abusers: a retrospective chart review. *Addict Behav* 1991; 16: 489-496.

[10] McCance-Katz, E. F., Carroll, K. M., and Rounsaville, B. J. Gender differences in treatment-seeking cocaine abusers--implications for treatment and prognosis. *Am J Addict* 1999; 8: 300-311.

[11] Dluzen, D. E. and Liu, B. Gender differences in methamphetamine use and responses: a review. *Gend Med* 2008; 5: 24-35.

[12] Hser, Y. I., Evans, E., and Huang, Y. C. Treatment outcomes among women and men methamphetamine abusers in California. *J Subst Abuse Treat* 2005; 28: 77-85.

[13] Brecht, M. L., O'Brien, A., von, Mayrhauser C., and Anglin, M. D. Methamphetamine use behaviors and gender differences. *Addict Behav* 2004; 29: 89-106.

[14] Semple, S. J., Grant, I., and Patterson, T. L. Female methamphetamine users: social characteristics and sexual risk behavior. *Women Health* 2004; 40: 35-50.

[15] Zweben, J. E., Cohen, J. B., Christian, D., Galloway, G. P., Salinardi, M., Parent, D., and Iguchi, M. Psychiatric symptoms in methamphetamine users. *Am J Addict* 2004; 13: 181-190.

[16] Derauf, C., LaGasse, L. L., Smith, L. M., Grant, P., Shah, R., Arria, A., Huestis, M., Haning, W., Strauss, A., Della, Grotta S., Liu, J., and Lester, B. M. Demographic and psychosocial characteristics of mothers

using methamphetamine during pregnancy: preliminary results of the infant development, environment, and lifestyle study (IDEAL). *Am J Drug Alcohol Abuse* 2007; 33: 281-289.

[17] Huber, A., Ling, W., Shoptaw, S., Gulati, V., Brethen, P., and Rawson, R. Integrating treatments for methamphetamine abuse: a psychosocial perspective. *J Addict Dis* 1997; 16: 41-50.

[18] Lauer, G. M. and Walker, B. D. Hepatitis C virus infection. *N Engl J Med* 7-5-2001; 345: 41-52.

[19] Centers for Disease Control and Prevention. HIV in the United Sates. *Centers for Disease Control and Prevention 2010.*

[20] Hunyady, B. [New treatment options of chronic hepatitis C virus infection.]. *Orv Hetil* 5-1-2011; 152: 887-897.

[21] Ghany, M. G., Strader, D. B., Thomas, D. L., and Seeff, L. B. *Diagnosis, management, and treatment of hepatitis C: an update. Hepatology* 2009; 49: 1335-1374.

[22] Chen, K. W., Banducci, A. N., Guller, L., Macatee, R. J., Lavelle, A., Daughters, S. B., and Lejuez, C. W. An examination of psychiatric comorbidities as a function of gender and substance type within an inpatient substance use treatment program. *Drug Alcohol Depend* 4-21-2011.

[23] Tidey, J. W., Mehl-Madrona, L., Higgins, S. T., and Badger, G. J. Psychiatric symptom severity in cocaine-dependent outpatients: demographics, drug use characteristics and treatment outcome. *Drug Alcohol Depend* 3-1-1998; 50: 9-17.

[24] Messina, N., Marinelli-Casey, P., Hillhouse, M., Rawson, R., Hunter, J., and Ang, A. Childhood adverse events and methamphetamine use among men and women. *J Psychoactive Drugs* 2008; Suppl 5: 399-409.

[25] Boyd, C. J. The antecedents of women's crack cocaine abuse: family substance abuse, sexual abuse, depression and illicit drug use. *J Subst Abuse Treat* 1993; 10: 433-438.

[26] Jantzen, K., Ball, S. A., Leventhal, J. M., and Schottenfeld, R. S. Types of abuse and cocaine use in pregnant women. *J Subst Abuse Treat* 1998; 15: 319-323.

[27] Volkow, N. D., Chang, L., Wang, G. J., Fowler, J. S., Franceschi, D., Sedler, M., Gatley, S. J., Miller, E., Hitzemann, R., Ding, Y. S., and Logan, J. Loss of dopamine transporters in methamphetamine abusers recovers with protracted abstinence. *J Neurosci* 12-1-2001; 21: 9414-9418.

[28] Paulus, M. P., Tapert, S. F., and Schuckit, M. A. Neural activation patterns of methamphetamine-dependent subjects during decision making predict relapse. *Arch Gen Psychiatry* 2005; 62: 761-768.

[29] Fitzgerald, N., Himmelgreen, D., Damio, G., Segura-Perez, S., Peng, Y. K., and Perez-Escamilla, R. Acculturation, socioeconomic status, obesity and lifestyle factors among low-income Puerto Rican women in Connecticut, U.S., 1998-1999. *Rev Panam Salud Publica* 2006; 19: 306-313.

In: Methamphetamines
Editors: J. Ornoy and X. He
ISBN: 978-1-62100-244-4

Chapter 7

IMPACT OF METHAMPHETAMINE ON DOPAMINE STORAGE AND RELEASE

Derick C. Davis, Andrew S. Sage and Dennis K. Miller*

Department of Psychological Sciences, Center for Translational Neuroscience, and Bond Life Science Center, University of Missouri, Columbia MO, US

ABSTRACT

Methamphetamine is a dangerous psychostimulant because of its high abuse potential and neurotoxic effects. This stimulant drug alters neurotransmitter storage, release and recycling in the central nervous system and increases levels of extraneuronal dopamine. The dopamine release is caused by methamphetamine's actions at the neuronal membrane-bound dopamine transporter and at the intraneuronal vesicular monoamine transporter. An understanding of how these monoamine transporters function and their interactions with methamphetamine to cause dopamine release is important to understand the pyschostimulant's behavioral and neurotoxic effects.

---

* Correspondence: Dennis K. Miller, Department of Psychological Sciences, University of Missouri, McAlester Hall, Columbia MO, 65210, USA. Tel: 573-884-8141, E-mail: millerden@missouri.edu.

INTRODUCTION

Methamphetamine is an extremely dangerous drug of abuse. A single use can result in extreme euphoria, but also presents a risk for neurotoxicity and neuronal death (Krasnova & Cadet, 2009). Methamphetamine produces its behavioral effects in the central nervous system through the vesicular monoamine transporter (VMAT) and the dopamine transporter (DAT)--proteins that regulate storage of the neurotransmitter dopamine. Dopamine is central to the methamphetamine's reinforcing (Olds & Milner, 1954; Robinson & Berridge, 1993, 2000) and toxic (Krasnova & Cadet, 2009) effects. Understanding the neurophysiology of methamphetamine's mechanism of action and key cellular transport proteins will help elucidate the dynamic effects this drug has on the central nervous system and consequently on behavior.

Neurotransmission could be considered a simple process with respect to the complex behaviors and actions it permits us to perform on a day-to-day basis (for a review on neuronal communication, Kalat, 2009; Kandel, Schwartz, & Jessell, 1995). Neurotransmission begins in the cytosol of the neuron with membrane depolarization and generation of an action potential. The action potential travels to the end of the axon—the terminal button—and leads to the release of signaling molecules called neurotransmitters from the neuron into the synapse, the area between neurons. This process of neurotransmission is depicted in Figure 1. Neurotransmitters diffuse across the synapse to bind postsynaptic receptors resulting in the transduction of neurochemical information.

Neurotransmission is a very dynamic, but discrete, process that is regulated within and outside the neuron *via* proteins called transporters (for review on transporters, Reith, 2010). Within the neuron, neurotransmitters are stored in vesicles. Vesicular transporters (e.g., VMAT2) shuttle neurotransmitter into the vesicles *via* an ion exchange process. Outside the neuron in the synapse, membrane-bound transporters remove neurotransmitter from the synapse *via* a sodium ion-dependent process (Yelin & Schuldiner, 2002). This process is referred to as reuptake. Drugs, such as methamphetamine, can alter chemical communication between neurons by changing neurotransmitter release and reuptake.

Methamphetamine produces a large and rapid increase in the extraneuronal concentration of dopamine and other monoamine neurotransmitters (e.g. serotonin and norepinephrine; Sulzer, Sonders, Poulsen, & Galli, 2005). This sudden increase in extraneuronal dopamine levels contributes to methamphetamine's profound effects on behavior. Figure 2 demonstrates the potency and efficacy of methamphetamine to increase extraneuronal dopamine levels in brain from an experiment in our laboratory. Rat brain (dorsal striatum) slices were loaded with [^{3}H]dopamine (radioactive— [^{3}H] — dopamine was used as a marker to trace dopamine movement into and out of the brain slices), placed in an automated superfusion system, and the [^{3}H]dopamine released (i.e. [^{3}H]overflow) was collected in 5-minute intervals. Methamphetamine (0.1 – 30 μM), within the concentration range observed in the central nervous system after *in vivo* treatment, was then applied. As depicted in Figure 2, methamphetamine produced a relatively rapid and concentration-dependent increase in extraneuronal [^{3}H]dopamine. The inset of Figure 2 depicts the time course of the experiment and the main panel depicts the amount of [^{3}H]dopamine released (i.e. area under the curve of the time course). An EC_{50} value of 6 μM was determined for methamphetamine to evoke [^{3}H]dopamine release. Our laboratory has shown that this process is affected by potential methamphetamine addiction pharmacotherapies (Rodvelt et al., 2011) and environmental toxins (Miller, Dopheide, Smith, & Casteel, 2005).

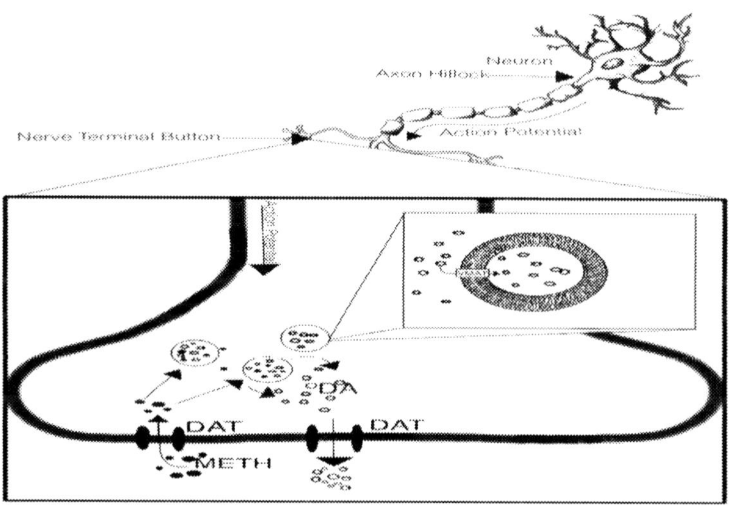

Figure 1. A schematic diagram of a dopamine neuron, with an enlargement of the terminal button. An action potential reaches the terminal button, where it leads to the release of neurotransmitter into the synapse. Neurotransmitter (dopamine, DA) storage is regulated within the neuron by vesicular transporters (VMAT) and outside the neuron by the DA transporter (DAT). Drugs, such as methamphetamine (METH) alter chemical communication by changing DAT and VMAT activity.

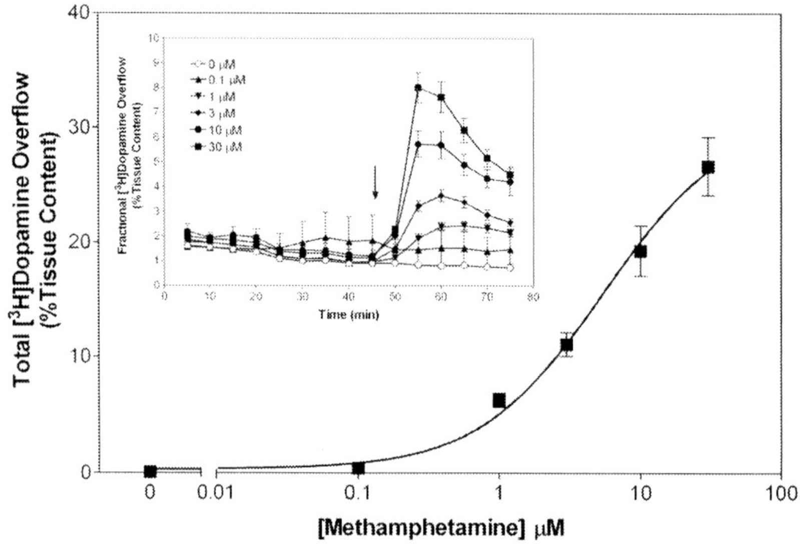

Figure 2. Methamphetamine produces a concentration-dependent increase in release of the neurotransmitter dopamine (i.e., [^{3}H]dopamine overflow). Rat brain (striatum) slices were loaded with [^{3}H]dopamine and methamphetamine (0.1 – 30 μM) was then added. Data in the main panel reflect the mean (±S.E.M.) total amount of neurotransmitter released (i.e., total [^{3}H]dopamine overflow) after the addition of methamphetamine. The inset reflects mean (±S.E.M.) neurotransmitter release as a time course (i.e., fractional [^{3}H] dopamine overflow). The arrow in the inset represents the addition of methamphetamine.

DOPAMINE

The neurotransmitter dopamine is a catecholamine that exists in both the central and the peripheral nervous system (for an overview, see Cooper, Bloom, & Roth, 2003). Dopamine has various roles within the body and functions as a chemical precursor for other catecholamine neurotransmitters (e.g., norepinephrine).

Methamphetamine's ability to suddenly and profoundly increase extraneuronal dopamine concentrations (Figure 2) is significant because dopamine is believed to contribute to stimulus salience and the development of drug "craving" that can follow repeated drug use (Robinson & Berridge, 1993, 2000). A stimulus (e.g. novelty, food, and methamphetamine) that induces dopamine release is perceived as rewarding and facilitates future stimulus recall and "wanting" of the stimulus. In addition to its role on stimulus salience and craving, dopamine has been suggested to be an underlying factor in the reinforcing properties of all abused drugs. Moreover, many studies have shown that dopamine is an essential component for methamphetamine toxicity (Krasnova & Cadet, 2009).

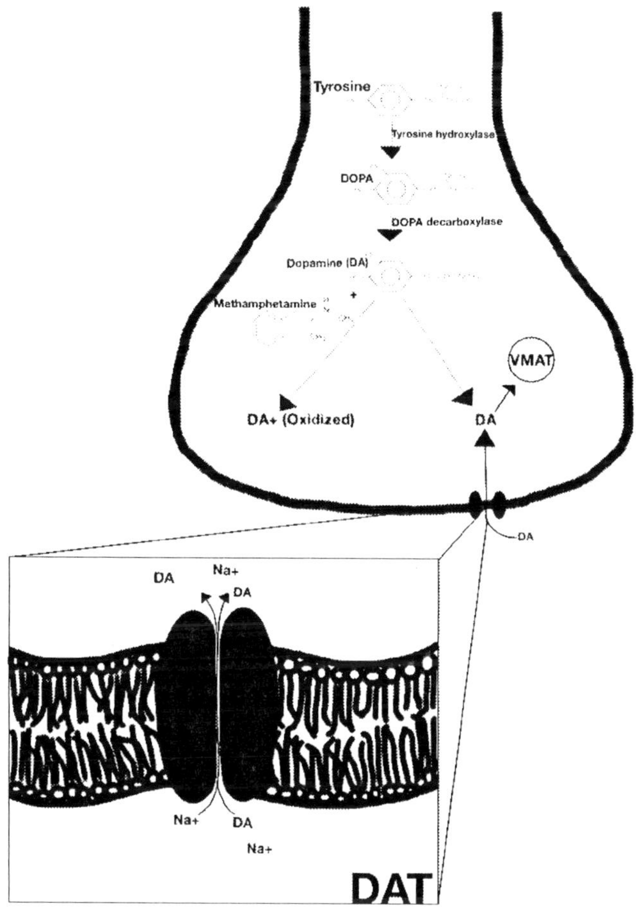

Figure 3. The terminal button of a dopamine (DA) neuron. DA is synthesized within the neuron from tyrosine and is stored in vesicles *via* the vesicular transporter (VMAT). Synaptic DA levels are regulated by the DA transporter (DAT), which works *via* coupling two sodium ions (Na^+). An impact of methamphetamine treatment is an increase in intraneuronal dopamine and its transformation to oxidized dopamine (DA+), which contributes to neurotoxicity.

NEUROTRANSMITTER CHEMISTRY

Dopamine's synthesis pathway is shown within a neuron in Figure 3 (for review of dopamine pharmacology, see Cooper et al., 2003). The "starting material" for dopamine synthesis is the amino acid L-tyrosine, which is converted to L-3,4-dihydroxyphenylalanine (L-DOPA) by the enzyme tyrosine hydroxylase. Tyrosine hydroxylase activity is a means of modulating the amount of dopamine synthesis and it is often used as a biological marker for dopamine neuron activity and toxicity. L-DOPA is converted to dopamine by the enzyme L-aromatic amino acid decarboxylase. The addition of more tyrosine has little effect on the rate of dopamine synthesis because tyrosine levels in the brain are above tyrosine hydroxylase's K_m value. However, addition of L-DOPA can substantially increase dopamine production because endogenous L-DOPA levels in the brain are low. As such, L-DOPA is used as a treatment for Parkinson's disease, to elevate the amount of dopamine in disease-affected nigrostriatal neurons. Dopamine metabolism within the neuron is under tight control by interneuronal enzymes. Once dopamine is transported back into the nerve terminal by DAT, the enzyme monoamine oxidase primarily converts dopamine into dihydroxyphenylacetic acid in the rodent brain and homovanillic acid in the human brain.

Dopamine Receptors

When dopamine is synthesized and released from presynaptic terminal buttons, it is received at pre-and postsynaptic D_1 and D_2 dopamine receptors. These receptors are distinguished by their effect on adenylate cyclase activity: D_1 dopamine receptors cause an increase of adenylate cyclase activity, while D_2 dopamine receptors decrease adenylate cyclase activity. These G-protein linked pathways mediate dopaminergic effects within the central nervous system, but they are not the only targets involved in dopamine's pharmacological action. For example, dopamine receptors can change inositol phosphate production and potassium (K^+) and calcium (Ca^{2+}) channel activity, which demonstrates the complexity of monoaminergic signaling pathways and the numerous effects that drugs, such as methamphetamine, can have on them.

Dopamine Transporter

In the central nervous system biogenic monoamine transporters, such as DAT, play a crucial role in regulating amine signaling and the neuronal neurotransmitter milieu (for review of transporters, see Reith, 2010). These transporters regulate monoamine neurotransmitters *via* reuptake from the synapse and terminate biogenic monoamine neurotransmission. The transporters utilize the energy of an asymmetrical ion gradient across the membrane to accumulate extraneuronal monoamines. The dopamine, norepinephrine, and serotonin transporters (DAT, NET, and SERT respectively) are responsible for regulating the extraneuronal movement of these monoamines and are the primary target for many psychotherapeutics and abused drugs, including methamphetamine.

Essential to these membrane transport systems and their ability to remove monoamines is the presence of K^+, sodium (Na^+), and chloride (Cl^-) ions. DAT, NET and SERT all utilize the asymmetrical ion distribution between the inside and outside of the neuron. To establish the asymmetrical ion distribution, energy from adenosine triphosphate (ATP) hydrolysis to adenosine diphosphate (ADP) is used. This energy is used to exchange three Na^+ ions out of the cell and two K^+ ions into the cell. The Na^+ and K^+ exchange, driven by the free energy release of a phosphate group being cleaved off of ATP, is depicted in Figure 4. Since the exchange of Na^+ and K^+ ions is uneven, an electrical gradient is created within the neuron. This negative membrane potential inside the neuron causes the efflux of Cl^- ions. These active ion gradients allow for an energetically-favorable uptake and accumulation of neurotransmitter within the neuron.

DAT, depicted in the bottom-left of Figure 3, is a member of the Na^+/Cl^--dependent membrane transporter family. DAT functions in the reuptake of dopamine into the terminal buttons of neurons. This membrane transporter utilizes an asymmetrical Na^+ concentration across the membrane (the Na^+ concentration is greater outside of the membrane) to drive the reuptake of dopamine. This process requires that two Na^+ ions be coupled along with one dopamine molecule for uptake into the terminal button. Although located in the terminal button, DAT is also expressed in regions outside the terminal button, where it may be involved with the reuptake of dopamine that has diffused away from the synapse. This suggests that initial inactivation of dopamine by removal from the synapse may be caused by diffusion.

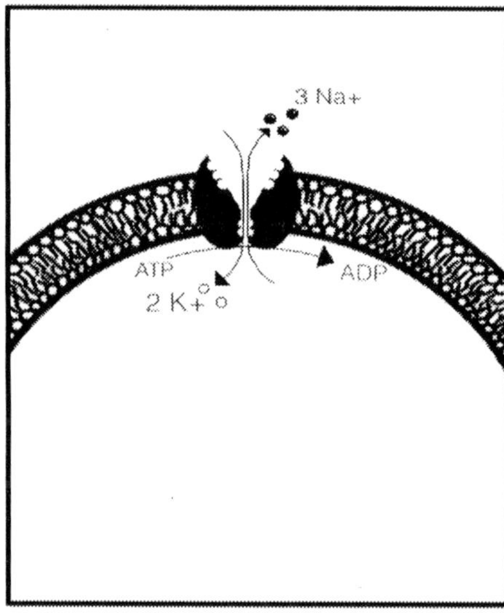

Figure 4. This neuronal membrane displays the sodium/potassium (Na^+/K^+) pump. Energy from adenosine triphosphate (ATP) hydrolysis to adenosine diphosphate (ADP) is used to maintain a Na^+ and K^+ gradient across the membrane.

Membrane transporters, such as DAT, are regulated themselves to cease monoamine transport. Methods by which transporters are regulated can be understood through analysis of their structures. DAT's amino acid sequence exhibits multiple consensus sites for interaction with intraneuronal proteins (e.g., domains on the cytosolic side of the membrane and protein kinases). DAT phosphorylation *via* protein kinases at these consensus sites results in changes in transporter activity, fusion with neurotransmitter-carrying vesicles and the membrane, endocytosis of the transporter, and transporter turnover (Ramamoorthy, 2002). Regulation of transporters may also occur through transporter interaction with other proteins *via* phosphorylation pathways (Blakely et al., 1998). Drugs that affect the structure of these monoamine transporters therefore affect the cell's ability to regulate the flow of monoamines back into the terminal button.

Vesicular Dopamine Storage

Vesicles are depicted as the large spheres within the terminal button in Figures 1 and 3 and "store" neurotransmitter, including dopamine. Figure 5 presents a schematic of a vesicle. Vesicular monoamine neurotransmitter transporters (indicated as VMAT in the figures) are similar in principle to DAT, but they function within the nerve terminal and traffic monoamines from cellular organelles to the border of the synapse and *vice versa* (for review of vesicular transporters, see Yelin & Schuldiner, 2002). Vesicular transporters utilize the energy released by ATP, and therefore use an asymmetrical ion gradient. The enzyme adenosine triphosphatase (ATPase) uses ATP hydrolysis to ADP to translocate hydrogen ions (H^+) into vesicles. The ATPase enzyme is depicted in Figure 5 as cleaving a phosphate group from ATP. This process drives H^+ across the membrane, which results in a positive and acidic (pH ≈ 5 – 5.6) environment in the vesicle. This H^+ electrochemical gradient then allows for the exchange of one H^+ from inside the vesicle for one neurotransmitter molecule outside the vesicle, through VMAT. H^+ ions are exchanged for dopamine molecules in the vesicle.

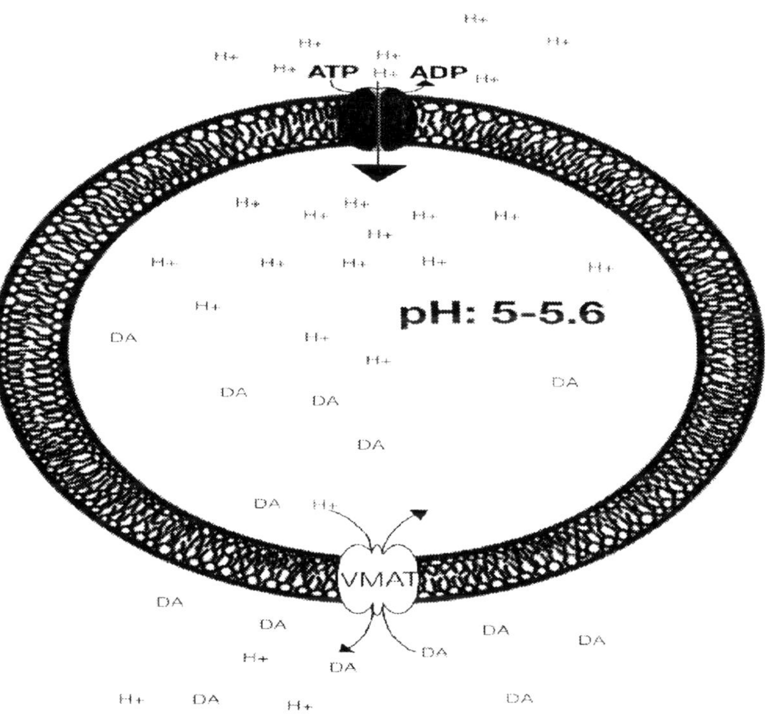

Figure 5. A neurotransmitter vesicle. Adenosine triphosphate (ATP) is hydrolyzed into adenosine diphosphate (ADP) to drive hydrogen ions (H^+) across the membrane, which results in an acidic environment in the vesicle. This H^+ electrochemical gradient then allows for the exchange of one H^+ from inside the vesicle for one dopamine (DA) molecule outside the vesicle through the vesicular neurotransmitter transporter (VMAT).

A specific vesicular transporter involved in methamphetamine action is VMAT. The action of VMAT and its role in biogenic amine transport can be better understood by examining when its activity is inhibited by drugs. (A common practice to understand a protein's function is to examine cellular activity when the protein of interest is inactive.) Two pharmacological VMAT inhibitors are reserpine and tetrabenazine (dihydro-tetrabenazine). Reserpine's effects are irreversible, which means its effects are only alleviated when new VMAT proteins replace those bound with reserpine. Tetrabenazine binding is reversible. Reserpine causes the depletion of monoamines, which gives a better understanding of VMAT's role when present in the cell. Competitive binding between reserpine and dopamine suggests the same site of recognition for both molecules (K_D values ≈ 30 pM) (Darchen, Scherman, & Henry, 1989). Radioligand studies with VMAT suggest separate binding sites for reserpine and tetrabenazine. This indicates that VMAT has two conformations, allowing for two mutually exclusive binding sites.

There are two VMAT isoforms—VMAT1 and VMAT2—and VMAT2 is more vital for methamphetamine function. The isoforms differ in their ligand binding profiles, with VMAT2 having greater sensitivity to substrates (e.g., dopamine) and tetrabenazine than VMAT1. This difference in affinity holds for methamphetamine, as VMAT2 has greater affinity for methamphetamine than VMAT1 has. VMAT1 resides primarily in non-neuronal cells and VMAT2 resides primarily in neurons.

Methamphetamine's Impact on Dopamine Storage and Release

Methamphetamine and other amphetamines (e.g., *d*-amphetamine and (-)-ephedrine) increase extraneuronal pools of dopamine (Figure 2) and it achieves this primarily through an interaction with VMAT2 and DAT. Briefly, methamphetamine blocks VMAT2 activity, which results in intra-neuronal pools of "free" dopamine. Methamphetamine induces the release of this dopamine pool into the synapse by "reversing" DAT activity.

Methamphetamine and the Dopamine Transporter

The hallmark of methamphetamine's effects on DAT is the reverse transport of cytosolic dopamine from the inside of the neuron out to the synapse (Sulzer et al., 2005). In other words, methamphetamine "reverses" the normal process of DAT from shuttling dopamine from the synapse into the cytosol to sending dopamine from the cytosol into the synapse. After methamphetamine administration (e.g., *via* inhalation or parenteral injection) enters the central nervous system through the blood-brain barrier and accumulates in the cytosol of the neuron *via* diffusion across the membrane or DAT uptake (Zaczek, Culp, & De Souza, 1991). Once inside the cytosol, methamphetamine causes dopamine reverse transport from within the terminal button. Sulzer and colleagues (1995) used a dopamine neuron from *Planorbis corneus*, a pond snail, to show amphetamine's ability to cause the reverse transport of dopamine, without blocking dopamine uptake. Discussed in an in-depth review, Sulzer and colleagues (1995) examined two hypotheses through which methamphetamine may bring about reverse transport of membrane transporters. Though many proposed hypotheses exist for a unified theory involving both of the hypothesized mechanisms, a conclusive mechanism remains to be determined.

The first hypothesis is known as facilitated exchange diffusion. This mechanism allows for a one-to-one exchange of catecholamine to methamphetamine between the nerve terminal button and the synapse. Since methamphetamine is a DAT substrate—a substance on which the transporter protein acts—it is taken up into the neuron by a substrate binding site on DAT. Methamphetamine is then released from within the cytosol *via* the substrate-binding site, which is now facing the inside of the neuron. Dopamine can then bind to the substrate binding site and cross the membrane into the synapse. The result of this process is an increase in the concentration of extraneuronal dopamine and the reverse transport by DAT. While this hypothesis is an attractive mechanism for transport reversal, it is not satisfactory to explain all of the details of dopamine release. For example, in the study conducted using *Planorbis cornes* (Sulzer et al., 1995) *d*-amphetamine was injected directly into the neuron terminal button--without any DAT uptake--and dopamine release was still observed.

In the second hypothesis discussed by Sulzer and colleagues (2005), methamphetamine causes dopamine release *via* channel-like transporter modes. Galli (1996, 1998) showed profound uncoupled ion movement across the membrane reminiscent of classical ion channels in neuronal membranes.

This conductance would allow for an exchange "rate" greater than the one dopamine molecule per one methamphetamine molecule, suggested by the previous facilitated exchange diffusion model. This mechanism has been observed with DAT (Sonders, Zhu, Zahniser, Kavanaugh, & Amara, 1997) and allows dopamine to travel across their concentration gradient, permitting very large release events.

Methamphetamine's mechanism to increase synaptic dopamine levels is not limited to DAT reverse transport. Schmitz and colleagues (2001) demonstrated that uptake inhibition also contributes to the increase in synaptic dopamine levels. (The psychostimulant cocaine increases synaptic dopamine levels by inhibiting neurotransmitter uptake (Reith, 2010).) *In vivo* methamphetamine treatment (i.e., parenteral injection) resulted in a decrease in the amount of dopamine uptake (i.e., a decrease in the V_{max} value for uptake kinetics) within one hour after stimulant injection, compared to vehicle treatment (Fleckenstein, Metzger, Wilkins, Gibb, & Hanson, 1997). This decrease in dopamine uptake was also observed with *in vitro* methamphetamine administration to striatal synaptosomes (Sandoval, Riddle, Ugarte, Hanson, & Fleckenstein, 2001).

Transporter phosphorylation has recently been shown to be a contributing factor to the effects of methamphetamine on DAT (Cervinski, Foster, & Vaughan, 2005). DAT phosphorylation and subsequent down-regulation would increase extraneuronal dopamine concentrations. Cervinski and colleagues (2005) reported a two-fold methamphetamine-induced increase in DAT phosphorylation in LLC-PK_1 cells. A similar increase was found in rat striatum following *in vivo* methamphetamine treatment (i.e., parenteral injection). This down-regulation of DAT was not thought to be mechanistically linked to methamphetamine's interactions with DAT. Down-regulation of DAT was still present when N-terminal phosphorylation sites were removed. Phosphorylation is thought to be associated with methamphetamine's effects on the efflux of dopamine to the synapse through DAT.

Methamphetamine and the Vesicular Transporter

While methamphetamine affects the membrane-bound DAT, its interaction with VMAT2 is also important for its efficacy and potency to increase synaptic dopamine levels. After methamphetamine enters into a neuron, it accumulates within the cytosol. Methamphetamine can then be transported into vesicles *via* diffusion or as a VMAT2 substrate (through a similar process to that described for DAT) and accumulate within the vesicle. The vesicular accumulation disrupts the H^+ gradient required for dopamine uptake into vesicles (Figure 5). As a result, there is increased cytosolic dopamine content. This "free pool" of dopamine is then available for release into the synapse *via* DAT, as described.

Methamphetamine's ability to increase dopamine levels within the neuron through VMAT2 inhibition is hypothesized to be due to methamphetamine's properties as a base ($pK_a \approx 9.8$; (Yogeeswari & Sriram, 2010). Vesicles maintain an acidic pH (Figure 5), which provides the H^+ gradient and energy needed to accumulate dopamine. Weak base compounds, such as methamphetamine, can bind free protons alkalinizing the existing acidic pH gradient. This increase in pH decreases the energy necessary to accumulate neurotransmitters within vesicles. The depletion or decrease of dopamine in the synaptic vesicles results in the redistribution of such molecules in the cytosol. This would increase the availability of transmitter for reverse transport by DAT. Methamphetamine-induced increases in cytosolic dopamine levels are important for the immediate reinforcing effects of the drug, which are related to rapid increases in synaptic dopamine (Gardner, 2011). Importantly, dopamine in the cytosol undergoes auto-oxidization (Hou et al., 2005)—a process in which oxygen is consumed and oxidative species are formed. Dopamine auto-oxidation generates hydrogen peroxide, dopamine quinones, superoxide radicals and hydroxyl radicals that can lead to oxidative stress and neuronal neurotoxicity (e.g., decrease in DAT protein and the density of terminal buttons, and neuronal death).

Pubill and colleagues (2005) showed that methamphetamine generated oxidative species in striatal synaptosomes with normal dopamine content, but did not generate oxidate species in dopamine-depleted synaptosomes (Pubill et al., 2005).

Evidence of dopamine-related toxicity can be seen in studies where dopamine synthesis inhibitors are used: Tyrosine hydroxylase inhibitors (e,g, α-methyl-p-tyrosine) decrease dopamine synthesis (Figure 3) and protect against methamphetamine-induced damage to striatal dopamine axons (Axt, Commin, Vosmer, & Seiden, 1990; Gibb & Kogan, 1979; Hotchkiss & Gibb, 1980; Schmidt, Garbutt, Wilkinson, & Ponder, 1985). Increasing L-DOPA levels (Figure 3) or preventing dopamine metabolism before methamphetamine treatment enhances stimulant-induced neurotoxicity (Gibb & Kogan, 1979; Schmidt et al., 1985).

Conclusion

In summary, the well-accepted mechanism through which methamphetamine exerts its greatest influence on behavior is by increasing synaptic dopamine levels. Methamphetamine produces a sudden and large increase in extraneuronal dopamine after direct application to neurons or by systemic administration (e.g., smoking, "snorting" or injecting the drug). Attempts to decrease methamphetamine use and dependence have focused on preventing the drug-induced increases in synaptic dopamine levels. Methamphetamine increases synaptic dopamine levels by altering the normal processes of neurotransmitter storage, release and recycling. The stimulant enters the neuron and creates a "free pool" of intraneuronal dopamine by inhibiting VMAT2 activity. Methamphetamine then "reverses" DAT, sending the dopamine into the synapse where it continues to interact with pre- and postsynaptic receptors influincing chemical signaling in pathways throughout the central nervous system.

Acknowledgment

Derick Davis' participation in research is supported by a grant from the University of Missouri College of Arts and Science Undergraduate Research Mentor Program. The authors' research on psychostimulant addiction is supported partially by a grant from the National Institute on Drug Abuse (DA028477) to John R. Lever, Susan Z. Lever and Dennis K. Miller at the University of Missouri.

References

Axt, K. J., Commins, D. L., Vosmer, G., & Seiden, L. S. (1990). α-Methyl-p-tyrosine pretreatment partially prevents methamphetamine-induced endogenous neurotoxin formation. *Brain Research*, *515*(1-2), 269-276.

Blakely, R. D., Ramamoorthy, S, Schroeter, S., Qian, Y., Apparsundaram, S., Galli, A, & DeFelice, L. J. (1998). Regulated phosphorylation and trafficking of antidepressant-sensitive serotonin transporter proteins. *Biological Psychiatry*, *44*(3), 169-178.

Cervinski, M. A., Foster, J. D., & Vaughan, R. A. (2005). Psychoactive substrates stimulate dopamine transporter phosphorylation and down-regulation by cocaine-sensitive and protein kinase C-dependent mechanisms. *The Journal of Biological Chemistry*, *280*(49).

Cooper, J., Bloom, F., & Roth, R. (2003). *The Biochemical Basis of Neuropharmacology*, New York: Oxford University Press.

Darchen, F., Scherman, D., & Henry, J. P. (1989). Reserpine binding to chromaffin granules suggests the existence of two conformations of the monoamine transporter. *Biochemistry*, *28*(4), 1692-1697.

Fleckenstein, A. E., Metzger, R. R., Wilkins, D. G., Gibb, J. W., & Hanson, G. R. (1997). Rapid and Reversible Effects of Methamphetamine on Dopamine Transporters. *Journal of Pharmacology and Experimental Therapeutics*, *282*(2), 834 -838.

Galli, A., Blakely, R. D., & DeFelice, L. J. (1996). Norepinephrine transporters have channel modes of conduction. *Proceedings of the National Academy of Sciences of the United States of America*, *93*(16), 8671-8676.

Galli, A., Blakely, R. D., & DeFelice, L. J. (1998). Patch-clamp and amperometric recordings from norepinephrine transporters: channel activity and voltage-dependent uptake. *Proceedings of the National Academy of Sciences of the United States of America*, *95*(22), 13260-13265.

Gardner, E. L. (2011). Addiction and brain reward and antireward pathways. *Advances in Psychosomatic Medicine*, *30*, 22-60.

Gibb, J. W., & Kogan, F. J. (1979). Influence of dopamine synthesis on methamphetamine-induced changes in striatal and adrenal tyrosine hydroxylase activity. *Naunyn-Schmiedeberg's Archives of Pharmacology*, *310*(2), 185-187.

Hotchkiss, A. J., & Gibb, J. W. (1980). Long-term effects of multiple doses of methamphetamine on tryptophan hydroxylase and tyrosine hydroxylase activity in rat brain. *The Journal of Pharmacology and Experimental Therapeutics*, *214*(2), 257-262.

Hou, Z., Sang, S., You, H., Lee, M.-J., Hong, J., Chin, K.-V., & Yang, C. S. (2005). Mechanism of action of (−)-epigallocatechin-3-gallate: Auto-oxidation–dependent inactivation of epidermal growth factor receptor and direct effects on growth inhibition in human esophageal cancer KYSE 150 Cells. *Cancer Research*, *65*(17), 8049 -8056.

Kalat, J. W. (2009). *Biological Psychology*. Belmont, CA: Wadsworth Publishing.

Kandel, E. R., Schwartz, J. H., & Jessell, T. M. (1995). *Essentials of neural science and behavior*. New York: McGraw-Hill Professional.

Krasnova, I. N., & Cadet, J. L. (2009). Methamphetamine toxicity and messengers of death. *Brain Research Reviews*, *60*(2), 379-407.

Miller, D. K., Dopheide, M. M., Smith, S. M., & Casteel, S. W. (2005). Dietary cadmium exposure attenuates D-amphetamine-evoked [^{3}H]dopamine release from striatal slices and methamphetamine-induced hyperactivity. *Pharmacology, Biochemistry, and Behavior*, *80*(4), 557-566.

Olds, J., & Milner, P. (1954). Positive reinforcement produced by electrical stimulation of septal area and other regions of rat brain. *Journal of Comparative and Physiological Psychology*, *47*(6), 419-427.

Pubill, D., Chipana, C., Camins, A., Pallàs, M., Camarasa, J., & Escubedo, E. (2005). Free radical production induced by methamphetamine in rat striatal synaptosomes. *Toxicology and Applied Pharmacology*, *204*(1), 57-68.

Ramamoorthy, S. (2002). Regulation of Monoamine Transporters: Regulated Phosphorylation, Dephosphorylation, and Trafficking. In M. E. A. Reith (Ed.), *Neurotransmitter Transporters*. Totowa, NJ: Humana Press.

Reith, M. E. A. (2010). *Neurotransmitter Transporters: Structure, Function, and Regulation.* Totowa, NJ: Humana Press.

Robinson, T. E., & Berridge, K. C. (1993). The neural basis of drug craving: an incentive-sensitization theory of addiction. *Brain Research. Brain Research Reviews*, *18*(3), 247-291.

Robinson, T. E., & Berridge, K. C. (2000). The psychology and neurobiology of addiction: an incentive–sensitization view. *Addiction*, *95*(8s2), 91-117.

Rodvelt, K. R., Oelrichs, C. E., Blount, L. R., Fan, K.-H., Lever, S. Z., Lever, J. R., & Miller, D. K. (2011). The sigma receptor agonist SA4503 both attenuates and enhances the effects of methamphetamine. *Drug and Alcohol Dependence*, *116*(1-3), 203-210.

Sandoval, V., Riddle, E. L., Ugarte, Y. V., Hanson, G R, & Fleckenstein, A. E. (2001). Methamphetamine-induced rapid and reversible changes in dopamine transporter function: an in vitro model. *Journal of Neuroscience*, *21*(4), 1413-1419.

Schmidt, G. H., Garbutt, D. J., Wilkinson, M. M., & Ponder, B. A. (1985). Clonal analysis of intestinal crypt populations in mouse aggregation chimaeras. *Journal of Embryology and Experimental Morphology*, *85*, 121-130.

Schmitz, Y., Lee, C. J., Schmauss, C., Gonon, F., & Sulzer, D. (2001). Amphetamine Distorts Stimulation-Dependent Dopamine Overflow: Effects on D2 Autoreceptors, Transporters, and Synaptic Vesicle Stores. *Journal of Neuroscience*, *21*(16), 5916 -5924.

Sonders, M. S., Zhu, S.-J., Zahniser, N. R., Kavanaugh, M. P., & Amara, S. G. (1997). Multiple Ionic Conductances of the Human Dopamine Transporter: The Actions of Dopamine and Psychostimulants. *Journal of Neuroscience*, *17*(3), 960 -974.

Sulzer, D., Chen, T. K., Lau, Y. Y., Kristensen, H., Rayport, S., & Ewing, A. (1995). Amphetamine redistributes dopamine from synaptic vesicles to the cytosol and promotes reverse transport. *Journal of Neuroscience*, *15*(5 Pt 2), 4102-4108.

Sulzer, D., Sonders, M. S., Poulsen, N. W., & Galli, A. (2005). Mechanisms of neurotransmitter release by amphetamines: A review. *Progress in Neurobiology*, *75*(6), 406-433.

Yelin, R., & Schuldiner, S. (2002). Vesicular Neurotransmitter Transporters: Pharmacology, Biochemistry, and Molecular Analysis. in Reith, M. E. A. (Ed.), *Neurotransmitter Transporters* Totowa, NJ: Humana Press.

Yogeeswari, P., & Sriram, D. (2010). *Medicinal Chemistry*. Upper Saddle River, NJ: Pearson Education.

Zaczek, R., Culp, S., & De Souza, E. B. (1991). Interactions of [^{3}H]amphetamine with rat brain synaptosomes. II. Active transport. *Journal of Pharmacology and Experimental Therapeutics*, *257*(2), 830-835.

In: Methamphetamines
Editors: J. Ornoy and X. He
ISBN: 978-1-62100-244-4

Chapter 8

PHARMACOLOGICAL ACTIONS OF *P*-HYDROXYAMPHETAMINE IN THE CENTRAL NERVOUS SYSTEM

Osamu Nakagawasai[1,*], Hiroshi Onogi[1,2], Satoru Mitazaki[1,3], Masato Hozumi[1], Koichi Tan-No[1], Yuichiro Arai[4], Tsuneaki Kikuchi[2] and Takeshi Tadano[1]

[1]Department of Pharmacology, Tohoku Pharmaceutical University, Sendai, Japan

[2]Faculty of Health Science, Tohoku Fukushi University, Sendai, Japan

[3]Laboratory of Forensic Toxicology, Faculty of Pharmacy, Takasaki University of Health and Welfare, Takasaki, Japan

[4]Tokyo Ariake University of Medical and Health Sciences, Tokyo, Japan

ABSTRACT

Methamphetamine (METH) and amphetamine (AMPH) are known to cause various behavioral changes, such as increased locomotor activity, stereotypy and prepulse inhibition (PPI) disruption, not only in humans

[*] Corresponding auther: Osamu Nakagawasai. Tel. and fax: +81-22-727-0123, E-mail address: osamun@tohoku-pharm.ac.jp; Address: Department of Pharmacology, Tohoku Pharmaceutical University, 4-4-1 Komatsushima, Aoba-ku, Sendai 981-8558, Japan.

but also in rodents. These behavioral changes are caused by releasing dopamine (DA), serotonin (5-HT) and noradrenaline (NA) within the brain. *p*-Hydroxyamphetamine (*p*-OHA), an active metabolite of both METH and AMPH, also has a number of pharmacological actions similar to those induced by drugs of abuse. Peripherally metabolized *p*-OHA does not easily cross the blood-brain barrier, but centrally metabolized *p*-OHA results in long-lasting stimulant effects. For example, intracerebroventricular administration of *p*-OHA induces a head-twitch response, indicating the involvement of the central serotonergic system. Also, *p*-OHA induces increased locomotor activity, indicating the involvement of the dopaminergic system. Moreover, *p*-OHA causes PPI disruption, indicating the involvement of the dopaminergic, serotonergic and noradrenergic systems. In in vitro experiments, *p*-OHA inhibits monoamine oxidase type A (MAO-A), thereby eliciting an increase in DA, NA and 5-HT levels. In this paper, we review the pharmacological properties and probable mechanisms of action of *p*-OHA.

INTRODUCTION

Methamphetamine (METH) and amphetamine (AMPH), indirect sympathomimetic compounds, cause their neurobehavioral effects, including anorexia, stimulation of physical performance, insomnia, euphoria, etc., by releasing dopamine (DA), serotonin (5-HT) and other neurotransmitters within the brain. Release of these neurotransmitters has been suggested to occur via two separate mechanisms: the redistribution of catecholamines from synaptic vesicles to the cytosol and induction of reverse transport of transmitters through their plasma membrane uptake carriers [1]. Other effects of AMPH, such as monoamine oxidase (MAO) inhibition, are also important for regulating extracellular catecholamine levels [2]. Substituted amphetamines, including methamphetamine (METH), methylphenidate, methylenedioxymethamphetamine (MDMA) and *p*-methoxyamphetamine (PMA), also play important medical and social roles in many cultures, exert profound effects on mental function and behavior, and can produce neurodegeneration and addiction [1].

METH and AMPH are metabolized to *p*-OHA in the periphery [3] and brain [4, 5], but peripherally metabolized *p*-OHA does not easily cross the blood-brain barrier [6]. In the brain, AMPH and METH are metabolized to *p*-OHA by the enzyme DA-L -hydroxylase [4, 5], and a further metabolite of *p*-OHA, *p*-hydroxynorephedrine (*p*-OHN), is formed by the enzyme in noradrenergic neurons [4, 5] in rodents (Figure 1). Interestingly, despite the rapid disappearance of AMPH and METH following administration, long-lasting accumulation of *p*-OHA is found in various brain regions including striatum, nucleus accumbens (NAc) and ventral tegmental area (VTA) [7, 8]. *p*-OHA has been shown to have a number of pharmacological actions, including causing psychostimulant-induced behaviors such as those induced by drugs of abuse [9-12]. In contrast, *p*-OHN does not cause these abnormal behaviors [13, 14]. These *p*-OHA-induced behaviors are due to the action of *p*-OHA itself on the central nervous systems and not from a further metabolite. For example, we have reported that intracerebroventricular (i.c.v.) administration of *p*-OHA induces 1) a head-twitch response (HTR), 2) hyperlocomotion and 3) prepulse inhibition (PPI) disruption in mice [14-17].

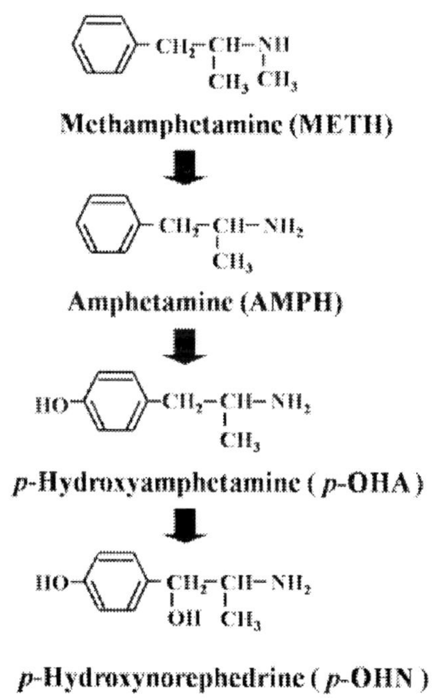

Figure 1. Main metabolic pathways of methamphetamine and amphetamine in humans.

1) HTR: The increase in monoamine content (especially, 5-HT) causes some abnormal behavioral pharmacology in mice, such as the HTR and the head-weaving response. It is known that head-weaving in animals is produced by excitation of 5-HT_{1A} receptors whereas the HTR is produced by excitation of 5-HT_{2A} receptors. The prefrontal cortex is an important locus for the production of the HTR [18]. During HTR behavior, mice rapidly shake their

head from side to side in a short period, typically less than half a second. It is known that administration of lysergic acid diethylamide (LSD) produces hallucinations in humans and that the HTR in mice is induced by administration of LSD. It is therefore thought that the HTR in mice represents hallucinations and can be used as a model of human hallucination. 2) Hyperlocomotion: The mesocorticolimbic DA pathways, particularly those projecting from the VTA (a DA cell body area) to the NAc (a DA terminal area), are known to be critical for the production of locomotor behaviors induced by psychomotor stimulants such as AMPH [19]. For example, locomotor sensitization is produced by administration of AMPH into the VTA but not by administration into the NAc [20]. Other reports have shown that AMPH-induced locomotor activity is, in part, mediated by DA release in the NAc, a brain region that is also critical for the rewarding effects of drugs [21].Studying the mechanisms underlying *p*-OHA-induced locomotor activity may provide insights into the subjectively rewarding effects of drugs in humans. 3) PPI disruption: PPI of the acoustic startle response (ASR) is a form of sensorimotor gating, defined as an inhibition of the startle reflex that occurs when the startling stimulus is preceded by a weak prestimulus [22]. Schizophrenia patients exhibit PPI impairment of the ASR, which is commonly interpreted as a sensorimotor gating deficit [23]. PPI is also diminished in rodents treated with psychotomimetic drugs such as AMPH, METH and phencyclidine [24-26]. The HTR, locomotor activity and PPI have been suggested to be relevant models for studying the pathophysiology of schizophrenia [22]. In addition, studying the mechanisms underlying *p*-OHA-induced abnormal behaviors provides insights into the withdrawal period following chronic administration of AMPH or METH [16]. Herein, we describe in detail the mechanisms underlying the HTR, hyperlocomotion and PPI deficits induced by *p*-OHA.

P-OHA-INDUCED HEAD-TWITCH RESPONSE

Direct application of *p*-OHA into the brain dose dependently induces the HTR in mice [27]. Treatment with diethyldithiocarbamate (DDC), an inhibitor of DA-β-hydroxylase (the enzyme responsible for further *p*-OHA metabolism), markedly enhances the frequency and duration of the *p*-OHA-induced HTR [28]. This is supported by our previous report [27] showing that the duration of the HTR is well correlated with the turnover rate of *p*-OHA following i.c.v. administration [29].

Table 1. Effects of serotonergic agents on *p*-OHA-induced head twitch response

Drug	Classification	Response
Diethyldithiocarbamate	Inhibitor of DA-β-hydroxylase	↑
Cyproheptadine	5-HT receptor antagonist	↓
Dimethothiazine	5-HT receptor antagonist	↓
p-Chlorophenylalanine	5-HT synthesis inhibitor	↓
Fluoxetine	Selective 5-HT uptake inhibitor	↓

The HTR induced by 5-HT-related agonists is inhibited by pretreatment with 5-HT_{2A} receptor antagonists [30]. We propose that the mechanism of *p*-OHA-induced HTR can be explained in terms of serotonergic neurons. The HTR is enhanced by the combined administration of *p*-OHA and 5-HT at the lowest doses of each compound that causes the HTR. In contrast, the HTR is markedly reduced by pretreatment with a 5-HT synthesis inhibitor such as cyproheptadine or dimethothiazine (Table 1, [15]) and by pretreatment with the selective 5-HT reuptake inhibitor, fluoxetine, at doses which do not cause the HTR [31]. From these findings, it is concluded that in order for *p*-OHA to induce the HTR it is necessary for 5-HT biosynthesis to increase and/or for 5-HT to be released from presynaptic neurons into the synaptic cleft.

It is well known that the HTR is enhanced by administration of HTR inducers in combination with MAO inhibitors [30]. The HTR induced by *p*-OHA is also enhanced by pretreatment with clorgyline, which is a potent MAO-A inhibitor, and it is suggested that MAO-A plays an important role in the occurrence of the HTR [27]. Our previous ex vivo study indicated that i.c.v. administration of *p*-OHA inhibits mouse brain MAO-A activity, however, *p*-OHN does not appreciably inhibit either MAO-A or MAO-B activity in mouse brain [9, 30]. These findings suggest that MAO-A inhibition is strongly involved in the HTR because 5-HT is inactivated by MAO-A but not by MAO-B. Following i.c.v. administration of *p*-OHA, the HTR lasts for 20-60 min, and the ex vivo inhibition of MAO-A activity by *p*-OHA is 20-40 min [9]. This time course of MAO-A inhibition by *p*-OHA ex vivo [9] is similar to the time course of the HTR induced by *p*-OHA [15, 32]. The correlation between the enzymatic activity (inhibition) and the behavioral response elicited by the injection of *p*-OHA seems very high. In addition, *p*-OHA greatly reduces 5-HT uptake into brain synaptosomes [33]. *p*-OHA accumulation in serotonergic nerve terminals increases MAO-A inhibition with an accompanying increase in 5-HT levels.

In summary, i.c.v. administered *p*-OHA is transported by the uptake system (5-HT transporter) into serotonergic nerve terminals. Thus, *p*-OHA taken up into serotonergic nerve terminals may elicit an increase in 5-HT levels by inhibiting MAO-A, and 5-HT is subsequently released into the synaptic cleft and/or neuronal cytosol from its store sites. This 5-HT release and its concomitant interaction with postsynaptic 5-HT_{2A} receptors are crucial steps in the induction of the HTR by *p*-OHA.

P-OHA-INDUCED HYPERLOCOMOTION

Administration of *p*-OHA (i.c.v.) significantly increases locomotor activity. However, a few studies have shown that i.p. injection of *p*-OHA does not change or decreases locomotor activity [34, 35], the reason for this discrepancy may be the route of administration. However, *p*-OHN did not influence locomotor activity in mice. Although both *p*-OHA and *p*-OHN inhibited MAO, *p*-OHA was shown to be more potent than *p*-OHN in inhibiting DA and 5-HT uptake from mouse forebrain homogenates [9]. Thus, the differences in our results with both compounds may be due to differences in their inhibitory effects on MAO, as well as on DA and 5-HT uptake.

As AMPH induces the release of monoamines, *p*-OHA has also been assumed to induce the release of neurotransmitters from presynaptic monoaminergic neurons. Previous reports have shown that the release of DA, NA and 5-HT can be induced by *p*-OHA [11, 36, 37]. In addition, previous studies have reported that central 5-HT and NA neural transmission is involved in the regulation of locomotor activity. For example, MDL100907, a selective 5-HT_{2A} antagonist, reversed the locomotor stimulant effects of AMPH in rats without having any effect on locomotor activity [38], and NA uptake inhibitors antagonized the locomotor-stimulant effect of AMPH [39]. Furthermore, as the DA-β-hydroxylase inhibitor DDC reduced NA levels [40-42], we used nomifensine, fluoxetine, or DDC treatment to determine whether *p*-OHA-induced hyperlocomotion is due to DA, 5-HT or NA release. *p*-OHA-induced locomotor activity was inhibited by pretreatment with nomifensine or haloperidol but not by pretreatment with fluoxetine or DDC (Table 2). These results indicate that DA neural transmission is one of the main factors involved in *p*-OHA-induced locomotor activity. *p*-OHA was suggested to be taken up into serotonergic as well as dopaminergic nerve terminals followed by DA release into the synaptic cleft [43]. The effects of nomifensine on *p*-OHA-induced hyperlocomotion could be due to its inhibition of *p*-OHA uptake into dopaminergic nerve terminals.

Table 2. Effects of dopaminergic and serotonergic agents on *p*-OHA-induced locomotor activity

Drug	Classification	Response
Haloperidol	DA receptor antagonist	↓
Nomifensine	DA reuptake inhibitor	↓
Fluoxetine	Selective 5-HT uptake inhibitor	±
Diethyldithiocarbamate	Inhibitor of DA-β-hydroxylase	±

To confirm the involvement of the dopaminergic system in *p*-OHA-induced locomotor activity, we focused on the mesocorticolimbic DA pathways, particularly those projecting from the VTA to the NAc, and tested the effects of *p*-OHA microinjection into the NAc on ambulation counts in rats. Local infusions of *p*-OHA into the NAc significantly increased ambulation counts and this ambulation was inhibited by pretreatment with nomifensine or haloperidol. Our results are consistent with previous findings showing that intra-NAc injections of AMPH produce increased locomotion [44]. Other reports have shown that AMPH-induced locomotor activity is blocked by DA receptor antagonists or by 6-hydroxydopamine lesions of DA nerve terminals in the NAc [45, 46]. Based on previous reports, our results indicate that the NAc may be important for the expression of locomotor activity induced by *p*-OHA.

We have previously shown that i.c.v. administration of *p*-OHA decreased striatal DA levels and its metabolite 3,4-dihydroxyphenylacetic acid (DOPAC), as well as inhibited DA uptake into the nerve endings and MAO activity [9, 43]. Cocaine and the DA transporter inhibitor GBR12909 increase locomotor activity because of the increased levels of synaptic DA which result from inhibition of DA reuptake [47]. In addition, administration of a MAO-inhibitor (for example, nialamide) alone to rodents induces little behavioral excitation [48]. It is also suggested that AMPH has inhibitory actions on MAO activity [49] and on the uptake of catecholamines at presynaptic nerve terminals [50]. Thus, *p*-OHA-induced hyperlocomotion could be due to an increase in DA levels in the NAc dopaminergic synaptic cleft which is attributable to the inhibitory effects of *p*-OHA on MAO and DA uptake.

Our research indicates that the central dopaminergic system is involved in *p*-OHA-induced locomotor activity in rodents and points to the NAc as an important site of action of *p*-OHA. However, *p*-OHA administration may also affect other NAc neurochemical systems involved in motor function, such as the glutamatergic and cholinergic systems.

P-OHA-INDUCED PREPULSE INHIBITION DISRUPTION

I.c.v. administration of *p*-OHA dose-dependently induced PPI disruption. *p*-OHA-induced PPI disruption was attenuated by pretreatment with both haloperidol (a predominantly D_2-blocking typical antipsychotic) and clozapine (a multi-receptor-blocking atypical antipsychotic) (Table 3). Haloperidol effects extended to all prepulse intensities and average PPI. Clozapine also attenuated PPI disruption over a wide range of prepulse intensities; however, clozapine effects were relatively weak compared to those of haloperidol. Clozapine has a highly complex pharmacological profile, with high affinity for a number of serotonin ($5\text{-}HT_{2A}$, $5\text{-}HT_{2C}$, $5\text{-}HT_6$, $5\text{-}HT_7$), dopamine (D_4), muscarinic (M_1, M_2, M_3, M_4, M_5), adrenergic (α_1- and α_2-subtypes) and other biogenic amine receptors [51]. Yamada [52] has pointed out that the ED_{50} value of the drugs (including typical antipsychotics) used to reverse apomorphine (a D_1 and D_2 agonist)-induced PPI disruption is significantly correlated with their affinity for the D_2 receptor but not for the D_1 receptor. As there is a difference in D_2 receptor affinity between haloperidol and clozapine, our results demonstrating the effects of these compounds indicate that the D_2 receptor may be involved in *p*-OHA-induced PPI disruption in mice. However, haloperidol also has affinity for the D_1, D_3 and D_4 receptors [51], and therefore we have to consider the possible involvement of these other DA receptor subtypes in the *p*-OHA-induced PPI disruption in mice. Furthermore, as *p*-OHA was suggested to be taken up into dopaminergic nerve terminals followed by DA release into the synaptic cleft [43] and because we have previously reported that *p*-OHA-induced hyperlocomotion is inhibited by a DA-reuptake inhibitor [14], we focused on the involvement of the central presynaptic or postsynaptic dopaminergic system in *p*-OHA-induced PPI disruption and investigated the effects of pretreatment with several dopaminergic agents. Regarding the effects of these DA receptor antagonists, *p*-OHA-induced PPI disruption was attenuated by pretreatment with L-741,626 (a selective D_2 receptor antagonist) and L-745,870 (a selective D_4 receptor antagonist), but not by SCH 23390 (a selective D_1 receptor antagonist) (Table 3). As described above, anti-DA agonist effects have been positively correlated with D_2 receptor affinity but not for D_1 receptors [52]. It has been proposed that DA dysfunction in schizophrenia includes both hyperfunction of subcortical D_2 and hypofunction of cortical D_1 systems [53]. The specific role of the D_3 receptor in the effects of DA agonists remains unclear because of limited selective ligand availability [54]. Our results demonstrating the effects of several DA receptor antagonists indicate that at least D_2 and D_4 receptors may be involved in *p*-OHA-induced PPI disruption in mice.

Table 3. Effects of dopaminergic and serotonergic agents on *p*-OHA-induced prepulse inhibition disruption

Drug	Classification	Attenuate/ineffective
Haloperidol	Typical antipsychotic	Attenuate
Clozapine	Atypical antipsychotic	Attenuate
SCH23390	Selective D_1 antagonist	Ineffective
L-741,626	Selective D_2 antagonist	Attenuate
L-745,870	Selective D_4 antagonist	Attenuate
6-Hydroxydopamine	Neurotoxin for DA neurons	Attenuate
GBR12909	DA-reuptake inhibitor	Ineffective
Ketanserin	$5\text{-}HT_{2A/2C}$ antagonist	Attenuate
MDL100,907	Selective $5\text{-}HT_{2A}$ antagonist	Attenuate
5,7-dihydroxytryptamine	Neurotoxin for 5-HT neurons	Attenuate
p- Chlorophenylalanine	5-HT synthesis inhibitor	Attenuate

It has been suggested that *p*-OHA is taken up into serotonergic as well as dopaminergic nerve terminals followed by DA release into the synaptic cleft [43]. Moreover, *p*-OHA-induced hyperlocomotion was inhibited by pretreatment with a DA-reuptake inhibitor [14]. Therefore, we used 6-OHDA (a neurotoxin which targets DA-containing neurons) to determine whether *p*-OHA-induced PPI disruptions are due to DA release into the synaptic cleft. Although it has been reported that 6-OHDA impaired PPI in rodents [55], we failed to induce PPI disruption with 6-OHDA at a dose of 40 μg/mouse. As a result, 6-OHDA lesions attenuated the extent of PPI disruption induced by *p*-OHA (Table 3). This is supported by a previous report that 6-OHDA lesions of the NAc in rats attenuated the ability of AMPH to disrupt PPI [56]. Our results indicate that selective blockade of either the D_2 or D_4 receptor subtype may prevent disruption of PPI induced by *p*-OHA via presynaptic DA release.

Haloperidol and clozapine have affinities for serotonergic (especially 5-HT_{2A}) receptors [51]. Therefore, we decided to investigate the involvement of the central serotonergic systems in *p*-OHA-induced PPI disruption. *p*-OHA-induced PPI disruption was attenuated by 5,7-dihydroxytryptamine (5,7-DHT, a neurotoxin which targets serotonin-containing neurons) and *p*-chlorophenylalanine (PCPA, a serotonin synthesis inhibitor) (Table 3). As both 5,7-DHT and PCPA were shown to reduce 5-HT levels [57-59], our results concerning the effects of presynaptic agents on *p*-OHA-induced PPI disruption indicate that increased 5-HT levels from presynaptic 5-HT nerve terminals are involved in *p*-OHA-induced PPI disruption. Ketanserin (a 5-$HT_{2A/2C}$ receptor antagonist) seemed to have a greater effect than MDL100,907 (both 5-HT_{2A} antagonists) on *p*-OHA-induced PPI disruption. Similarly, PCPA seemed to have a greater effect than 5,7-DHT (both reduce 5-HT levels). There is speculation that these differences in efficacy may be due to the properties of the pretreatment agents with respect to specificity for serotonergic and noradrenergic transmitter systems. Ketanserin has affinity for 5-$HT_{2A/2C}$ receptors, but also binds with less potency to the α_1 receptor [60], whereas MDL100,907 is a more selective 5-HT_{2A} receptor antagonist than ketanserin [61]. Given that these previous studies suggest that compounds with noradrenergic actions via α_1 receptors as well as compounds with serotonergic actions via 5-HT_{2A} receptors might be effective antipsychotics [51], our results indicate that compounds which have both serotonergic and noradrenergic actions might be more effective in attenuating *p*-OHA-induced PPI disruption than selective serotonergic compounds such as MDL100,907 or 5,7-DHT. Our preliminary data showed that prazosin, an α_1 receptor antagonist, attenuates *p*-OHA-induced PPI disruption. It was suggested that noradrenergic systems could play a role in central gating mechanisms. Our research indicates that *p*-OHA induces PPI disruptions via presynaptic DA and 5-HT release.

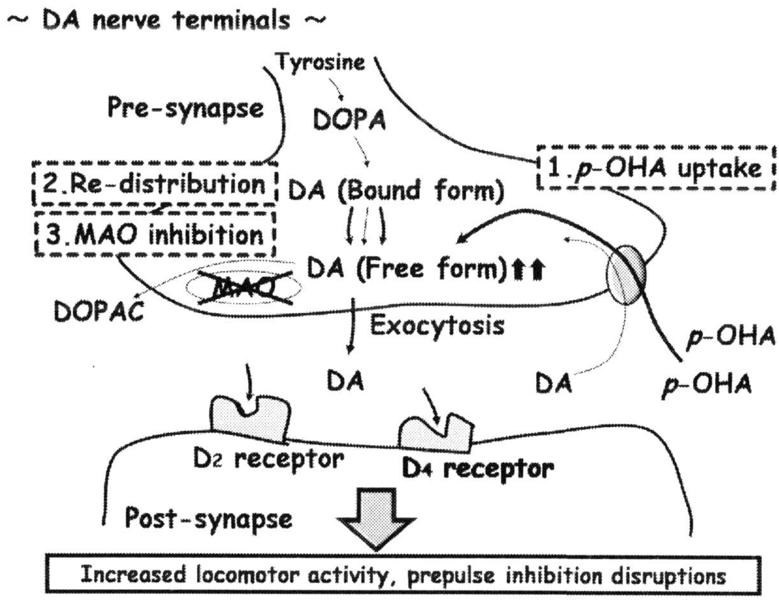

Figure 2. Proposed schematic representation of the interaction between *p*-OHA and DA nerve terminals. Bold texts and arrows indicate proposed mechanism of *p*-OHA action.

The mechanism of hyperlocomotion and PPI disruption by p-OHA is schematically shown in Figure 2. An explanation of the induction mechanism of *p*-OHA-induced behaviors may be that neurotransmitters are accumulated in dopaminergic and serotonergic nerve terminals via the DA and 5-HT uptake systems. Following this accumulation, brain DA and 5-HT levels could be further increased by inhibition of intraneuronal MAO activity. Increased DA and 5-HT levels in the neuron are released from nerve endings into the synaptic cleft by nerve stimulus. The increased DA and 5-HT levels in the synaptic cleft would consequently cause activation of postsynaptic D_2, D_4 and 5-HT_{2A} receptors. Our results indicate that blockade of the D_2, D_4 and 5-HT_{2A} receptor subtype may prevent *p*-OHA-induced behaviors. This exploration of the unique properties of *p*-OHA may help to elucidate psychostimulant actions in the central nervous system with the view to ultimately clarifying schizophrenia-relevant pathogenesis.

References

[1] D. Sulzer, M. S. Sonders, N. W. Poulsen and A. Galli, *Prog. Neurobiol.* 75, 406 (2005).

[2] M. C. Scorza, C. Carrau, R. Silveira, G. Zapata-Torres, B. K. Cassels and M. Reyes-Parada, *Biochem. Pharmacol.* 54, 1361 (1997).

[3] M. Y. Law, M. H. Slawson and D. E. Moody, *Drug Metab. Dispos.* 28, 348 (2000).

[4] M. Goldstein and J. F. Contrera, *J. Biol. Chem.* 237, 1898 (1962).

[5] M. Goldstein and B. Anagnoste, *Biochimica et Biophysica Acta* 107, 166 (1965).

[6] A. Lindenbaum, K. Marcher, J. Wepierre and Y. Cohen, *Archives Internationales de Pharmacodynamie et de Therapie* 215, 168 (1975).

[7] A. Jori and S. Caccia, *J. Pharm. Pharmacol.* 26, 746 (1974).

[8] C. M. Kuhn, S. M. Schanberg and G. R. Breese, *Biochem. Pharmacol.* 27, 343 (1978).

[9] Y. Arai, S. K. Kim, H. Kinemuchi, T. Tadano, S. E. Satoh, N. Satoh et al. *J. Neurochem.* 55, 403 (1990).

[10] D. F. Dougan, S. L. Labrie, P. D. Paull, P. H. Duffield and D. N. Wade, *Gen. Pharmacol.* 17, 453 (1986).

[11] L. M. Kaminskas, R. J. Irvine, P. D. Callaghan, J. M. White and P. Kirkbride, *Psychopharmacology* 160, 155 (2002).

[12] L. L. Simpson, *J. Pharmacol. Exp. Ther.* 213, 504 (1980).

[13] S. Sakurada, *Folia Pharmacol Jpn* 71, 779 (1975).

[14] H. Onogi, M. Hozumi, O. Nakagawasai, Y. Arai, S. Ishigaki, A. Sato, S. Furuta, F. Niijima, K. Tan-No and T. Tadano, *Psychopharmacology* 208, 323 (2010).

[15] T. Tadano, S. Satoh and K. Kisara, *Jpn J. Pharmacol.* 41, 519 (1986).

[16] H. Onogi, O. Nakagawasai, K. Tan-No, S. Mitazaki, A. Sato, K. Nakaya. F. Niijima, Y. Arai, T. Kikuchi, T. Tadano, *Behav. Brain Res.* 214, 349 (2010).

[17] H. Onogi, O. Nakagawasai, A. Sato, S. Mitazaki, K. Nakaya, K. Watanabe, F. Niijima-Yaoita, K. Tan-No, Y. Arai, T. Kikuchi and T. Tadano, *Behav Brain Res.* in press.

[18] D. L. Willins and H. Y. Meltzer, *J. Pharmacol. Exp. Ther.* 282, 699 (1997).

[19] P. Vezina, *Neurosci Biobehav Rev* 27, 827 (2004).

[20] M. Cador, Y. Bjijou and L. Stinus, *Neuroscience* 65, 385 (1995).

[21] G. Di Chiara and A. Imperato, *Proc Natl Acad Sci USA* 85, 5274 (1988).

[22] M. A. Geyer, K. Krebs-Thomson, D. L. Braff and N. R. Swerdlow, *Psychopharmacology* 156, 117 (2001).
[23] N. R. Swerdlow, D. L. Braff, N. Taaid and M. A. Geyer, *Arch Gen Psychiatry* 51, 139 (1994).
[24] S. Arai, K. Takuma, H. Mizoguchi, D. Ibi, T. Nagai, K. Takahashi, et al. *Neuropsychopharmacology* 33, 3164 (2008).
[25] R. S. Mansbach, M. A. Geyer and D. L. Braff, *Psychopharmacology* 94, 507 (1988).
[26] R. S. Mansbach and M. A. Geyer, *Neuropsychopharmacology* 2, 299 (1989).
[27] T. Tadano, S. Satoh, N. Satoh, K. Kisara, Y. Arai, S.K. Kim et al. *J. Pharmacol. Exp. Ther.* 250, 254 (1989).
[28] S. Satoh, N. Satoh, T. Tadano and K. Kisara, *Res. Commun. Sub. Abuse* 6, 213 (1985).
[29] W. A. Taylor and F. Sulser, *J. Pharmacol. Exp. Ther.* 185, 620 (1973).
[30] O. Nakagawasai, Y. Arai, S. Satoh, N. Satoh, M. Neda, M. Hozumi, R. Oka, H. Hiraga and T. Tadano, *Neurotoxicology* 25, 223 (2004).
[31] K. Oyama, T. Tadano, K. Kisara, Y. Arai and H. Kinemuchi, *Jpn J. Pharmacol.* 49, 335 (1989).
[32] T. Tadano, S. Satoh, N. Satoh, K. Kisara, Y. Arai and H. Kinemuchi, *Neuropharmacology* 26, 1463 (1987).
[33] Y. Arai, S. K. Kim, H. Kinemuchi, T. Tadano, S. Satoh, N. Satoh et al. *Neurochem. Int.* 17, 587 (1990).
[34] R. H. Bauer, *Pharmacol. Biochem. Behav.* 13, 155 (1980).
[35] P. J. Bushnell, *Pharmacol. Biochem. Behav.* 25, 161 (1986).
[36] A. K. Cho, J. F. Fischer and J. C. Schaeffer, *Biochem. Pharmacol.* 26, 1367 (1977).
[37] L. A. Matsuda, G. R. Hanson and J. W. Gibb, *J. Pharmacol. Exp. Ther.* 251, 901 (1989).
[38] P. C. Moser, P. M. Moran, R. A. Frank and J. H. Kehne, *Behav. Brain Res.* 73, 163 (1996).
[39] T. D. Tyler and R. E. Tessel, *Psychopharmacology* 69, 27 (1980).
[40] G. G. Collins, *J. Pharm. Pharmacol.* 17, 526 (1965).
[41] W. J. Chang, C. R. Barb, R. R. Kraeling, G. B. Rampacek and J. T. Wright, *J. Anim. Sci.* 73, 1147 (1995).
[42] M. Gaval-Cruz, J. P. Schroeder, L. C. Liles, M. A. Javors and D. Weinshenker, *Pharmacol. Biochem. Behav.* 89, 556 (2008).
[43] Y. Arai, S. K. Kim, H. Kinemuchi, T. Tadano, K. Oyama, N. Satoh N and K. Kisara, *Brain Res. Bull.* 27, 81 (1991).

[44] P. Vezina and J. Stewart, *Brain Res.* 516, 99 (1990).
[45] E. M. Joyce and G. F. Koob, *Psychopharmacology* 73, 311 (1981).
[46] P. Vezina P, *J. Neurosci.* 16, 2411 (1996).
[47] A. J. Mcgeehan, P. H. Janak and M. F. Olive, *Psychopharmacology* 174, 266 (2004).
[48] H. Kuribara, *Pharmacol. Biochem. Behav.* 56, 9 (1997).
[49] H. Kuribara and S. Tadokoro, *Jpn. J. Pharmacol.* 33, 1127 (1983).
[50] B. A. McMillen, *Trends Pharmacol. Sci.* 4, 429 (1983).
[51] B. L. Roth, D. J. Sheffler and W. K. Kroeze, *Nat. Rev. Drug Discov.* 3, 353 (2004).
[52] S. Yamada, *Nihon Shinkei Seishin Yakurigaku Zasshi* 20, 131 (2000).
[53] J. K. Seamans and C. R. Yang, *Prog. Neurobiol.* 74, 1 (2004).
[54] R. J. Ralph, G. B. Varty, M. A. Kelly, Y. M. Wang, M. G. Caron, M. Rubinstein, D. K. Grandy, M. J. Low and M. A. Geyer, *J. Neurosci.* 19, 4627 (1999).
[55] M. Bubser and M. Koch, *Psychopharmacology* 113, 487 (1994).
[56] N. R. Swerdlow, R. S. Mansbach, M. A. Geyer, L. Pulvirenti, G. F. Koob and D. L. Braff, *Psychopharmacology* 100, 413 (1990).
[57] S. Jha, R. Rajendran, J. Davda and V. A. Vaidya, *Brain Res.* 1075, 48 (2006).
[58] Y. Maruyama, G. Hayashi, S. E. Smits and A. E. Takemori, *J. Pharmacol. Exp. Ther.* 178, 20 (1971).
[59] M. F. Snape, M. I. Colado and A. R. Green, *Pharmacol. Toxicol.* 74, 40 (1994).
[60] K. P. Bøgesø, J. Arnt, V. Boeck, A. V. Christensen, J. Hyttel and K. G. Jensen, *J. Med. Chem.* 31, 2247 (1988).
[61] N. M. Barnes and T. Sharp, *Neuropharmacology* 38, 1083 (1999).

In: Methamphetamines
Editors: J. Ornoy and X. He

ISBN: 978-1-62100-244-4

Chapter 9

DEPENDENCE, PSYCHIATRIC SYMPTOMS AND COGNITIVE IMPAIRMENT INDUCED BY METHAMPHETAMINE USE DISORDER

Kazufumi Akiyama*[*], *Atsushi Saito*, *Go Kuratomi*, and *Yosefu Arime
Department of Biological Psychiatry and Neuroscience
Dokkyo Medical University School of Medicine

ABSTRACT

Since the early 1950s, Japan has experienced three major epidemics of methamphetamine (METH) use. Increasing prevalence rates in the general population for METH use have recently been reported from other pan-pacific nations. METH use disorder still imposes a burden on current mental health in Japan. Strong cravings are a feature of METH use disorder, as many patients find difficulty in refraining from re-using it during abstinence. Recent functional neuroimaging studies show that the craving for METH may be associated with reduced activity in some brain areas involved in decision making. Most noticeably, the paranoid-hallucinatory state resembling paranoid schizophrenia has been regarded as a hallmark of METH-induced psychosis. The current diagnosis of

[*] Corresponding author: Kazufumi Akiyama, MD.Ph.D. Department of Biological Psychiatry and Neuroscience, Dokkyo Medical University School of Medicine. E-mail address: kazufuak@dokkyomed.ac.jp.

substance-induced psychotic disorder is defined by DSM-IV as a prototypical intoxication-induced or withdrawal-associated psychotic episode. Even the substance-induced psychotic disorder that occurs in the context of substance use disorder has not been sufficiently recognized. Although METH-induced psychosis usually resolves rapidly with the cessation of stimulant use, a subset of currently abstinent METH-dependent patients develop protracted psychosis even after long-term abstinence. Several reports indicate that protracted METH psychosis is more likely to occur among METH abusers with a pre-morbid schizoid/schizotypal personality trait and those with a family history of schizophrenia among first-degree relatives. Further study is needed concerning the role of pre-morbid vulnerability to protracted METH psychosis. Recent studies have also noted a high rate of the life time prevalence of affective symptoms such as depression, suicide attempts, and impulsivity in METH abusers. Caution should be exercised in treating female METH abusers who have a higher risk of suicide than male METH abusers. Studies using positron emission tomography demonstrated that exposure to METH induces a robust change in the neurotransmission of dopamine and serotonin neurons. These studies have shown that the reductions of dopamine and serotonin transporter are associated with cognitive impairment and enhanced impulsivity in patients with METH-induced psychosis.

INTRODUCTION

Methamphetamine (METH) is a potent psychostimulant with high dependence liability. Since the early 1950s, Japan has experienced three major epidemics, termed 1st epidemic (1945-1956), 2nd epidemic (1971-1995) and 3rd epidemic (1995-present) (Tatetsu 1963; Sato et al 1983; Iwanami et al 1994; Akiyama 2006; Akiyama et al 2011; Wada 2011). During the last decade, the prevalence of METH use has increased at an escalating pace in pan-pacific countries (Kulsudjarit 2004; Maxwell JC and Rutkowski 2008). METH use disorder imposes a burden on mental health in Japanese society. This short review introduces the current situation of METH use in Japan and discusses some problems involving craving, psychiatric symptoms and cognitive impairment induced by METH use disorder.

History of METH Abuse in Japan: General Population, Arrestees, Psychiatric Hospitals

The Nationwide Mental Hospital Survey on Drug-related Psychiatric Disorders, which have been conducted every other year by the National Center for Neurology and Psychiatry (NCNP) since 1976, shows that METH remains a major abused psychoactive drug causing a high rate of psychiatric sequelae. METH has ranked the highest among all illicit drugs causing psychotic symptoms, in that nearly half of drug-related patients compelled to be admitted involuntarily to mental hospitals have been METH users (Wada 2011). Approximately 11, 000- 14,000 offenders who use METH against the Stimulant Control Law are arrested every year, representing about 80 % of all drug-related arrestees in Japan. However, this figure represents only a small fraction of the total METH users in Japan, since lifetime prevalence of METH use is estimated to be 0.4 % of the general population according to an NCNP questionnaire survey which has been conducted for randomly selected subjects at ages higher than 15 years (Wada 2011). Thus, the spread of METH use in the general population features the current status of METH use in Japan. More seriously, 59% and 42% of METH users spend periods exceeding five and ten years, respectively, suggesting that a large number of METH users are repeat offenders.

The epidemics of METH use in Japan have mingled to some extent with substance use disorders involving other illicit drugs, accounting for the complex history of multi-drug use in Japan. The onset of use disorders of volatile solvents and cannabis took place during the 2nd METH epidemic. During this period, arrestees who violated the Poisonous and Deleterious Substance Law by using volatile solvents outnumbered those who used METH (Wada 2011). Although the number of arrestees using volatile solvents decreased remarkably in the 3rd METH epidemic, volatile solvents have since ranked the highest in terms of life time prevalence of any kind of substance use; life time prevalence of volatile solvents is estimated to be 1.5 - 2.0 % of the general population (Wada 2011). Cannabis is another popular illicit drug in Japan, and cannabis-related arrestees outnumbered those of volatile solvent-related arrestees in 2006 (Wada 2011). The current life time prevalence of cannabis use is estimated to be 0.8 % of the general population (Wada 2011). Many METH users who exhibit METH psychosis use other illicit substances as well as METH. Approximately 55% and 35% of METH-related patients treated in mental hospitals use concomitantly with volatile solvents and cannabis, respectively. It is considered quite likely that teenagers using volatile solvents transferred to METH use in the 2nd METH epidemic, indicating that preceding volatile solvents play a key role in preparing a gateway for METH use disorder (Miura et al, 2006; Wada 2011). It is plausible that the high rate of lifetime prevalence of volatile solvent use in the current general population in Japan reflects the overwhelming number of users of these substances in the 2nd METH epidemic. We recently reported that patients who had used a volatile solvent prior to METH in their teenage years showed a significantly earlier onset of METH use than the rest of patients who had not used volatile solvents. (18.4 ±3.5 for volatile solvent–using group vs. 22.5 ±6.6 years old for non-volatile solvent–using group, Akiyama et al 2011).

Craving for METH Use

Environmental factors, such as an injection needle and bootleg place, are learned as cues which are associated with strong craving for METH. These cues are also called conditioned incentive stimuli (Robinson and Berridge 1993). Although precise assessment of the intensity of cravings for METH-associated cues is difficult and fell behind that of psychiatric symptoms of METH psychosis, a newly developed method using a visual analogue scale .enables quantitative measurement of the intensity of craving (Hartz et al 2001; Galloway et al 2009). These studies provide evidence that METH-associated craving can predict subsequent probability of re-use leading to relapses (Hartz et al 2001; Galloway et al 2009).

The empirical fact that a number of patients with METH use disorder and accompanying cognitive dysfunction are prone to re-using METH upon exposure to drug-associated cues suggests that certain impairment of decision-making may underlie such liabilities to re-use. A functional MRI study using a decision-making task shows that brain activity in the right insula and inferior parietal cortex is significantly lower in patients who relapsed one year later than those maintaining abstinence (Paulus et al 2005). These brain areas are involved in decision-making which takes precedence over long-term benefit, suggesting that the dysfunction in these brain regions may contribute to relapses. There is a report showing correlation between the intensity of craving for METH use and depressive symptoms during abstinence (Nakamura et al 2008).

SYMPTOMS OF METH PSYCHOSIS

As the last decade has seen that the prevalence of METH use disorder increased at an escalating pace worldwide (Kulsudjarit 2004; Maxwell JC and Rutkowski 2008), the high rate of psychiatric sequelae resulting from METH use disorder has been recognized on a global scale. It is well documented that METH is a potent catecholamine/serotonin releaser. The acute psychotropic effect of METH is marked by euphoria, talkativeness, grandiosity, enhanced drive for sexual activity, and reduced requirement of sleep. With repeated use, these hedonic responses to METH are gradually replaced by anhedonia, such as general fatigue, avolition, and other unpleasant experiences. Paranoid-hallucinatory states rarely occur as an acute reaction to METH in those who have not used it previously However, a very large dose can induce a confusional state which manifests as robust intoxication features consisting of a clouding of the consciousness, extreme fear and paranoid-hallucination. Latency to the emergence of a paranoid-hallucinatory state during repeated regimens depends on amount, route of administration (intravenous injection vs. inhalation), purity of the drug, and surrounding circumstances of where it is used (Matsumoto et al 2002). We found that the average latency to the emergence of the first frank psychotic episode was 4 years (Akiyama et al 2011) which is comparable to the mean latency of 4.4 years for abusers who self-injected METH intravenously in a previous Japanese report (Matsumoto et al 2002). These data indicate that late-onset adaptation in neural circuitry underlies the manifestation of METH psychosis

METH psychosis is typically characterized by a paranoid-hallucinatory state resembling paranoid schizophrenia (Sato et al 1983, Iwanami et al 1994, Akiyama 2006, Akiyama et al 2011, Chen et al 2003; Chen et al 2005; McKetin et al 2006, Mahoney et al 2008). Delusions in METH psychosis include delusions of reference, persecution, and of mind-reading. Most delusions in patients with METH psychosis are concerned with their family or people who they know in everyday life. Some patients feel as if his or her neighbors are laughing at him or her. They hear voices that insult them or order them to kill themselves. Besides auditory hallucinations, vivid visual hallucinations are sometimes experienced. Auditory hallucinations sometimes are paired with visual hallucinations. For instance, some patient may feel as if a scary face in front of him or her speaking directly to them. Bizarre tactile hallucinations, such as a feeling of worms crawling beneath the skin, are occasionally experienced

Affective symptoms are also important in METH psychosis as a precipitating factor associated with suicide risk. In fact, patients with METH psychosis often exhibit depression/suicide attempts (Kalechstein et al 2000; Lin et al 2004, Zweben et al 2004, Yen et al 2005; Glasner-Edwards et al 2008a, 2008b), and impulsive/violent behaviors (Kalechstein et al 2000;Chen et al 2003, Lin et al 2004). Multiple factors have been implicated in suicidal ideation in adolescent METH abusers (Yen et al 2005). Gender difference should be considered of high priority in this regard, since several studies have consistently demonstrated that female patients are more susceptible to the risk of suicide than male patients (Lin et al 2004; Zweben et al 2004). We confirmed a high rate of suicide attempts in female patients with METH psychosis (Akiyama et al 2011). Precipitated aggression is another important affective symptom in METH psychosis. A neuroimaging study showed that serotonin transporters in the anterior cingulate cortex and anterior orbital cortex are robustly reduced in patients with METH use disorder who show symptoms of enhanced aggression (Sekine et al 2006).

Protracted METH Psychosis

The current diagnosis of substance-induced psychotic disorder is based on DSM-IV criteria which assume a prototypical intoxication-induced or withdrawal-associated psychotic episode (American Psychiatric Association). Specifically, amphetamine-induced psychotic disorder is narrowly defined as an intoxication-induced psychotic episode in DSM-IV (American Psychiatric Association). This concept follows the classical view proposed by Connell (1958), and cannot account for a psychotic episode in the context of substance use disorder only. (Matsumoto et al 2002; Macketin et al 2006; Farrell et al 2002; Mathias et al 2008). Given that psychotic episode can occur in subjects with METH use disorder (Matsumoto et al 2002; Macketin et al 2006; Farrell et al 2002), METH psychosis should rather be defined as a broad spectrum of drug-associated psychotic disorder, as previously suggested (Mathias et al 2008). Japanese investigators saw that a subset of currently abstinent METH-dependent patients develop protracted psychosis even after a long-term cessation of stimulant use (Tatetsu 1963, Sato et al 1983, Iwanami et al 1994, Akiyama 2006, Akiyama et al 2011). Previous literatures noted that the prevalence of abstinent METH users whose psychotic symptoms lasted for a minimum period of one month was about 4% - 26% on average among METH abusers in Japan (Iwanami et al 1994) and Taiwan (Chen et al 2003; Chen et al

2005; Lin et al 2004). In support of these data, Kittirattanapaiboon et al (2010) reported recently that Thailand METH patients who had been hospitalized previously were divided into those with a single episode of psychosis (52.6%) and those with a chronic course of psychosis (38.8%).

Incarcerated subjects provided an advantage for demographic studies of METH psychosis: confirmed and supervised abstinence during imprisonment (Akiyama 2006, Akiyama et al 2011; Farrell et al 2002). Thus, incarcerated patients with METH psychosis might contribute to an understanding of the trajectory of their severe psychiatric symptoms during long-term abstinence. We recently reported protracted METH psychosis after a supervised abstinence period of 13.5 ±10.6 months (mean ±S.D.) during imprisonment in eighty incarcerated female Japanese patients who had used METH for 12.0 ±7.5 years (mean ±S.D.) (Akiyama et al 2011). Many conditions are necessary to explain the protracted psychosis with METH use disorder. It is plausible that they represent the extremity in continuity with more benign conditions in terms of symptom severity and duration. We do not have exact knowledge regarding how such a long-term use of METH contributes to refractory psychotic symptoms. It cannot be excluded that pre-morbid psychiatric disorders may precipitate protracted psychosis. Therefore, causality of protracted METH psychosis should be considered in the context of interaction between long-time exposure to METH and personal history indicative of early cognitive predisposition.

Chen et al (2003) reported comparison of demographic features between patients with METH-induced psychosis (MIP) and those with no experience with psychotic symptoms (MNP). They demonstrated that MIP subjects started METH use earlier, used larger METH dosages, and had pre-morbid schizoid/schizotypal personality traits more frequently than MNP subjects (Chen et al 2003). The onset of amphetamine use before the age of 16 years was also reported to be a risk factor precipitating psychosis in prisoners in England and Wales (Farrell et al 2002). Moreover, Chen et al (2003) reported that the pre-morbid schizoid/schizotypal personality trait was more frequently associated with MIP, which lasted for an abstinence of over one month than MIP which resolved within one month. The same investigators also reported that patients with MIP lasting for more than 1 month abstinence were associated with significantly higher morbid risk of schizophrenia in their first-degree relatives than those with MIP resolving less than one month and those with MNP (Chen et al 2005).

Patients with protracted METH psychosis are usually diagnosed as having schizophrenia as well as METH use disorder in Western countries according to the current DSM-IV criteria (American Psychiatric Association). Several reports indicate that pre-existing schizophrenia may precipitate chronic METH psychosis (McKetin et al 2006; Zweben et al. 2006). However, these investigators also suggest that the comorbidity cannot be verified only by assessing cross-sectional symptoms (McKetin et al 2006; Zweben et al. 2006).

Enduring Cognitive Dysfunction in METH Use Disorder

Several lines of evidence indicate that patients with METH use disorder have cognitive dysfunction, which impairs their social function and adherence to medical therapy. Thus, these patients maintaing in abstinence show a delayed response time in the Stroop test, indicating that their ability to focus their attention on a target is compromised (Salo et al 2002). A functional MRI study revealed that patients with METH dependence after 2- 4 month abstinence show reduced activity in the frontal cortex when undergoing the Stroop test (Salo et al 2009). It is hypothesized that neural cell injury is involved in cognitive dysfunction associated with METH use (Rose and Grant 2008). It has been reported, even in long-term abstinence, dopamine transporters in the basal ganglia of patients with METH dependence is reduced in proportion to cognitive decline (Volkow et al 2001).

Treatment of Craving for METH Use and of METH Psychosis

Strong craving for METH re-use shall be a treatment target in METH use disorder. Although very few medications which inhibit the craving for METH are available, it was recently reported that bupropion reduced acute METH-induced subjective effects and reduced cue-induced craving (Newton et al 2006). It is presumably advisable to treat patients manifesting METH psychosis with second-generation antipsychotics as recommended in previous case-reports (Mirsa 1997, Mirsa 2000, Satter 2004). However, there is no systematic study which compares different antipsychotic prescriptions to reveal efficacious medication for METH psychosis, nor is there an algorithm which proposes a treatment strategy. Furthermore, patients with METH psychosis exhibit such complex cross-sectional symptoms that there is a need to develop appropriate and efficient pharmacotherapy for the required dosages of antidepressants and mood stabilizers.

References

Akiyama K, Saito A, Shimoda K. Chronic methamphetamine psychosis after long-term abstinence in Japanese incarcerated patients. *Am J Addict* 20:240-249, 2011.

Akiyama K. Longitudinal clinical course following pharmacological treatment of methamphetamine psychosis which persists after long-term abstinence. *Ann N Y Acad Sci* 1074:125-134, 2006.

American Psychiatric Association. *Diagnostic and Statistical Manual of Mental Disorders,* Fourth Edition, Text Revision. Washington, DC. American Psychiatric Association; 2000.

Chen C-K, Lin S-K, Sham PC, Ball D, Loh E-W, Hsiao C-C et al. Pre-morbid characteristics and co-morbidity of methamphetamine users with and without psychosis. *Psychol Med.* 33:1407-1414, 2003.

Chen C-K, Lin S-K, Sham PC, Ball D, Loh E-W, Murray RM. Morbid risk for psychiatric disorder among the relatives of methamphetamine users with and without psychosis. *Am J Med Genetics Part* B136B:87-91, 2005

Connell PH. *Amphetamine psychosis,* Maudsley Monographs No5, London, 1958.

Farrell M, Boys A, Bebbington P, Brugha T, Coid J, Jenkins R,et al.. Psychosis and drug dependence: Results from a national survey of prisoners. *Brit J Psychiatry* 181:393-398, 2002.

Galloway GP, Singleton EG, the Methamphetamine Treatment Project Corporate Authors. How long does craving predict use of methamphetamine? Assessment of use one to seven weeks after the assessment of craving. *Substance Abuse* 26:63-79, 2009.

Glasner-Edwards S, Mooney LJ, Marinelli-Casey, P. Hillhouse M, Ang A, Rawson R. et al. Risk factors for suicide attempts in methamphetamine-dependent patients. *Am J Addict.* 17:24-27, 2008a.

Glasner-Edwards S, Mooney LJ, Marinelli-Casey, P., Hillhouse M, Ang A, Rawson R et al. Identifying methamphetamine users at risk for major depressive disorder: findings from the methamphetamine treatment project at three year follow-up. *Am J Addict.* 17:99-102, 2008b.

Hartz DT, Frederick-Osbourne SL, Galloway GP. Craving predicts use during treatment for methamphetamine dependence: a prospective, repeated measures, within-subject. *Drug Alcohol Dependence* 63:269-276, 2001.

Iwanami A, Sugiyama A, Kuroki N, Toda S, Kato N, Nakatani Y et al. Patients with methamphetamine psychosis admitted to a psychiatric hospital in Japan. A preliminary report. *Acta Psychiatr Scand* 89:428-432, 1994.

Kalechstein AD, Newton TF, Longshore D, Anglin MD, van Gorp WG, Gawin FH. Psychiatric comorbidity of methamphetamine dependence in a forensic sample. *J Neuropsychiatry Clin* Neurosci 12:480-484, 2000.

Kittirattanapaiboon P, Mahatnirunkul S, Booncharoen H, Thummawomg P, Dumrongchai U, Chutha W. Long-term outcomes in methamphetamine psychosis patients after first hospitalization. *Drug Alcohol Rev* 29:456-461, 2010.

Kulsudjarit K. Drug problem in Southeast and Southwest Asia. *Ann N.Y. Acad Sci* 1025:446-457, 2004.

Lin S-K, Ball D, Hsiao C-C, Chiang Y-L, Ree S-H, Chen C-K. Psychiatric comorbidity and gender differences of persons incarcerated for methamphetamine abuse in Taiwan. *Psychiatry Clini Neurosci* 58:206-212, 2004.

Mahoney JJ, Kalechstein AD, De La Garza R, Newton TF. Presence and persistence of psychotic symptoms in cocaine- versus methamphetamine-dependent participants. *Am J Addiction* 17:83-98, 2008.

Mathias S, Lubman DI, Hides L. Substance-induced psychosis: A diagnostic conundrum. *J Clin Psychiatry* 69:359-367, 2008.

Matsumoto T, Kamijo A, Miyakawa T, Endo K, Yabana T, Kishimoto H et al. Methamphetamine in Japan: the consequences of methamphetamine abuse as a function of route of administration. *Addiction.* 97:809-817, 2002.

Maxwell JC and Rutkowski BA. The prevalence of methamphetamine and amphetamine abuse in North America: a review of the indicators, 1992-2007. *Drug Alcohol Rev* 27:229-235, 2008.

McKetin R, McLaren J, Lubman DI, Hides L.. The prevalence of psychotic symptoms among methamphetamine users. *Addiction.* 101:1473-1478, 2006.

Misra L, Kofoed L. Risperidone treatment of methamphetamine psychosis. *Am J Psychiatry.* 154:1170, 1997.

Misra LK, Kofoed L, Oesterheld JR, Richards G.A. Olanzapine treatment of methamphetamine psychosis. J Clin Psychopharmacol. 20:393-394, 2000.

Miura H, Fujiki M, Shibata A, Ishikawa K. Prevalence and profile of methamphetamine users in adolescents at a juvenile classification home. *Psychiatry Clin Neurosci* 60:352-357, 2006.

Nakamura H, Chang L, Closk C, Jiang C, Alicata D, Haning W. Association between psychiatric symptoms and craving in methamphetamine users. *Am J Addiction* 17:441-446, 2008.

Newton TF, Roache JD, De La Garza R II, Fong T, Wallace CL, Li S-H et al. Bupropion reduces methamphetamine-induced subjective effects and cue-induced craving. *Neuropsychopharmacology* 31:1537-1544, 2006.

Paulus MP, Tapert SF, Schuckit MA. Neural activation patterns of methamphetamine-dependent subjects during decision making predict relapse. *Arch Gen Psychiatry* 62:761-768, 2005.

Robinson TE, Berridge KC. The neural basis of drug-craving: An incentive-sensitization theory of addiction. *Brain Res Rev* 18:247-291, 1993.

Rose ME, Grant JE: Pharmacotherapy for methamphetamine dependence: A review of the pathophysiology of methamphetamine addiction and the theoretical basis and efficacy of pharmacotherapeutic interventions. *Ann Clin Psychiatry* 20:145-155, 2008.

Salo R, Nordahl TE, Possin K, Leamon M, Gibson DR, Galloway GP et al: Preliminary evidence of reduced cognitive inhibition in methamphetamine-dependent individuals. *Psychiatry Res* 111:65-74, 2002.

Salo R, Ursu S, Buonocore MH, Leamon MH, Carter C. Impaired prefrontal cortical function and disrupted adaptive cognitive control in methamphetamine abusers: A functional magnetic resonance imaging study. *Biol Psychiatry* 65:706-709, 2009.

Sato M, Chen C-C, Akiyama K, Otsuki S. Acute exacerbation of paranoid psychotic state after long-term abstinence in patients with previous methamphetamine psychosis. *Biol Psychiatry* 18:429-440, 1983.

Sattar SP, Bhatia SC, Petty F. Potential benefits of quetiapine in the treatment of substance dependence disorders. *J Psychiatry Neurosci* 29:452-457, 2004.

Sekine Y, Ouchi Y, Takei N, Yoshikawa E, Nakamura K, Futatsubashi M et al. Brain serotonin transporter density and aggression in abstinent methamphetamine abusers. *Arch Gen Psychiatry* 63:90-100, 2006.

Tatetsu S. Methamphetamine psychosis. *Folia Psychiatr Neurol Jpn. Suppl* 7:377-380, 1963.

Volkow ND, Chang L, Wang G-J, Fowler JS, Keonido-Yee M, Franceschi D et al. Association of dopamine transporter reduction with psychomotor impairment in methamphetamine abusers. *Am J Psychiatry* 158:377-382, 2001.

Wada K. The history and current state of drug abuse in Japan. *Ann N.Y. Acad. Sci.* 1216:62-72, 2011.

Yen C-F, Shieh B-L. Suicidal ideation and correlates in Taiwanese adolescent methamphetamine users. *J Nerv Ment Dis.* 193:444-449, 2005.

Zweben JE, Cohen JB, Christian D. Galloway GP, Salinardi M, Parent D et al.. Psychiatric symptoms in methamphetamine users. *Am J Addict.* 13:181-190, 2004.

INDEX

D

E

F

G

H

I

J

K

L

M

N

Q

R

S

T